Further praise for *Sleep Well on the Autism Spectrum*:

'This book is absolutely packed with useful current information that reflects research into sleep disorders. Although it is an excellent resource for professionals, the flow charts are well-designed and represent good practice to keep the focus for parents. The rating system for different interventions is particularly good. This will definitely become a resource frequently employed in Scottish Autism's sleep counselling services.'

— *Alan Somerville, Chief Executive, Scottish Autism*

by the same author

Sleep Difficulties and Autism Spectrum Disorders
A Guide for Parents and Professionals
Kenneth J. Aitken
ISBN 978 1 84905 259 7
eISBN 978 0 85700 550 2

Dietary Interventions in Autism Spectrum Disorders
Why They Work When They Do, Why They Don't When They Don't
Kenneth J. Aitken
ISBN 978 1 84310 939 6
eISBN 978 1 84642 860 9

An A–Z of Genetic Factors in Autism
A Handbook for Parents and Carers
Kenneth J. Aitken
ISBN 978 1 84310 679 1
eISBN 978 0 85700 388 1

of related interest

The Complete Guide to Asperger's Syndrome
Tony Attwood
ISBN 978 1 84310 495 7 (hardback)
ISBN 978 1 84310 669 2 (paperback)
eISBN 978 1 84642 559 2

SLEEP WELL
ON THE AUTISM SPECTRUM

How to recognise common sleep difficulties,
choose the right treatment, and get you
or your child sleeping soundly

KENNETH J. AITKEN

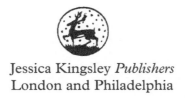

Jessica Kingsley *Publishers*
London and Philadelphia

Peter's Social Story outline on page 58 adapted from Moore 2004 with kind permission from John Wiley and Sons © 2004.
Box B1 on page 93 adapted from Picchietti and Picchietti 2008 with kind permission from Elsevier © 2008.

First published in 2014
by Jessica Kingsley Publishers
73 Collier Street
London N1 9BE, UK
and
400 Market Street, Suite 400
Philadelphia, PA 19106, USA

www.jkp.com

Library of Congress Cataloging in Publication Data
A CIP catalog record for this book is available from the Library of Congress

British Library Cataloguing in Publication Data
A CIP catalogue record for this book is available from the British Library

ISBN 978 1 84905 333 4
eISBN 978 0 85700 668 4

Printed and bound in Great Britain

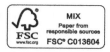

*To my wonderful wife Ros, and to Natasha and Chantal,
the two daughters who have taught us, in their very different
ways, a lot of what we know about the vagaries of sleep*

ACKNOWLEDGEMENTS

Over the years, I have known and worked with hundreds of families affected by ASD. I have also had the privilege of lecturing to and learning from families and clinicians around the world – including Japan, Australia, Qatar, the USA, Canada, Brazil, South Africa, Israel, France, Spain, Portugal, Germany, Sweden, Denmark, Greece, Poland, Romania, Eire and throughout the UK.

I am grateful to the many families whose problems have taught me what I know today, to all of the clinicians and researchers who have generously shared their work with me and to all the colleagues and friends who have commented on drafts of this evolving manuscript and helped to make it as good as it is. Any errors and inaccuracies are of course entirely of my own making.

DISCLAIMER

This volume has been carefully produced and edited. Nevertheless, the author, editors and publishers do not warrant that the information is entirely free from errors. The reader is advised to bear in mind that all statements, data, illustrations and details may contain inadvertent inaccuracies.

The problem you might be dealing with and where to start

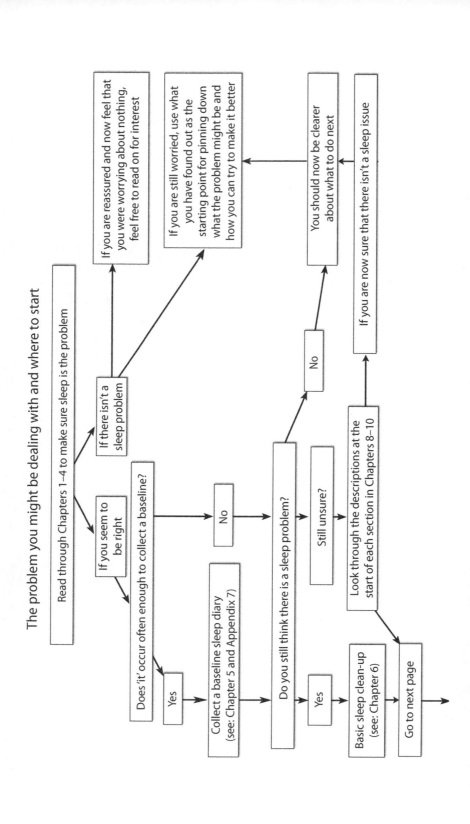

Read through Chapters 1–4 to make sure sleep is the problem

If there isn't a sleep problem

If you are reassured and now feel that you were worrying about nothing, feel free to read on for interest

If you are still worried, use what you have found out as the starting point for pinning down what the problem might be and how you can try to make it better

If you seem to be right

Does 'it' occur often enough to collect a baseline?

Yes

No

Collect a baseline sleep diary (see: Chapter 5 and Appendix 7)

Do you still think there is a sleep problem?

Yes

No

Still unsure?

You should now be clearer about what to do next

If you are now sure that there isn't a sleep issue

Look through the descriptions at the start of each section in Chapters 8–10

Basic sleep clean-up (see: Chapter 6)

Go to next page

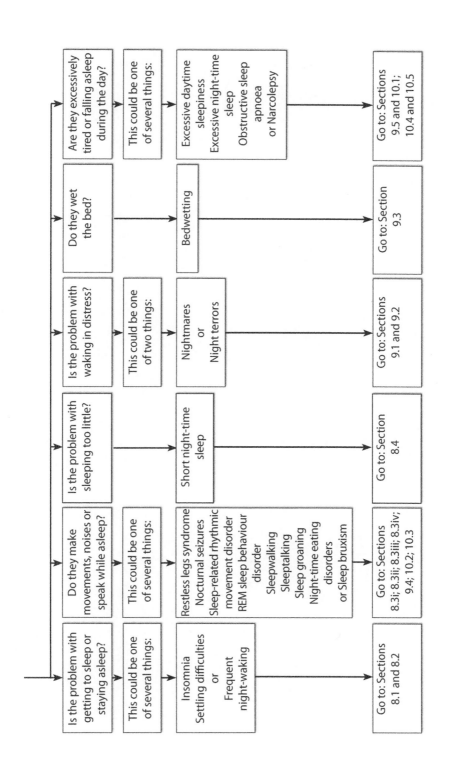

Is the problem with getting to sleep or staying asleep?	Do they make movements, noises or speak while asleep?	Is the problem with sleeping too little?	Is the problem with waking in distress?	Do they wet the bed?	Are they excessively tired or falling asleep during the day?
This could be one of several things:	This could be one of several things:		This could be one of two things:		This could be one of several things:
Insomnia Settling difficulties or Frequent night-waking	Restless legs syndrome Nocturnal seizures Sleep-related rhythmic movement disorder REM sleep behaviour disorder Sleepwalking Sleeptalking Sleep groaning Night-time eating disorders or Sleep bruxism	Short night-time sleep	Nightmares or Night terrors	Bedwetting	Excessive daytime sleepiness Excessive night-time sleep Obstructive sleep apnoea or Narcolepsy
Go to: Sections 8.1 and 8.2	Go to: Sections 8.3i; 8.3ii; 8.3iii; 8.3iv; 9.4; 10.2; 10.3	Go to: Section 8.4	Go to: Sections 9.1 and 9.2	Go to: Section 9.3	Go to: Sections 9.5 and 10.1; 10.4 and 10.5

CONTENTS

List of Figures, Tables and Boxes

Figures

Tables

Boxes

INTRODUCTION

What this book is about

Anyone struggling to get to sleep or to cope with someone else's sleep problems knows only too well the serious effects they can have. A good night's sleep can make even the biggest problems seem easier to deal with (and they usually are after a decent sleep), while regular nights of broken sleep can make every small molehill seem like a mountain.

This is a book about the various sleep issues seen in people with ASD. I have tried to explain the best approaches to use, and how to find the right help when sleep problems are causing difficulty or distress, making this as simple as possible while trying to keep it practical. I have used a 'recipe book' layout to show the approaches that seem to work best with each type of problem, how easy and practical they should be to carry out and, based on published studies, how successful they can be.

There is no off-the-shelf approach that works for 'sleep problems', but there are many solutions and a variety of possible problems. You need to work out what your problem is and what might work before trying to work on it. For most sleep problems there are approaches with a good chance of helping, and some of the broad outlines of what to do are the same, but the specific details of what might work are different.

Some problems will have no 'tried-and-tested' approach. When previous work is unhelpful in deciding what to do, you need to do some problem-solving of your own to work out a possible solution. You just have to think about this as your special problem and use the problem-focused approach outlined here to work out what might help.

Every problem is unique, and for some it will be easier to see possible things you could try than for others.

The main focus here is on describing the most common sleep issues, explaining how they might be helped, describing the approach or approaches that usually work best, and what is involved.

It can be easier to follow through with any approach if you understand what you are dealing with, and are familiar with some of the reasons that trying to improve things can be so important. To help you understand each problem, I have described how to assess it, given a brief description of the problem and a summary of what we know about it. Where possible, I also review the evidence on what can help.

The term 'ASD' is used widely throughout this book. It is an acronym that stands for Autistic Spectrum Disorders. The term ASD, introduced in the Diagnostic and Statistical Manual of Mental Disorders DSM-5 system revision, replaced the earlier terms used to describe all people who would have been diagnosed with Autistic Disorder (autism), Asperger's Disorder, Childhood Disintegrative Disorder (CDD) or Pervasive Developmental Disorder-Not Otherwise Specified (PDD-NOS). DSM-5 was adopted by the American Psychiatric Association in May 2013.

To help you to understand how difficult the different approaches we discuss might be, each section has a simple rating system using four icons. These show:

- where additional costs might be involved (the more £ signs, the more expensive)

- how difficult it is to do (the more hammers, the more effort involved)

- how likely it is to work (the more Rosettes, the more successful it is reported to be)

and:

- any possible problems or issues (the more clouds, the more likely it is to have difficulties; a sun means there are no reported problems).

These icons are shown below:

	Cost of doing it	Difficulty doing it	Chances of it working	Possible problems
Least ↑ ↓ Greatest	£ £ £ £ £ £ £ £ £ £ £ £ £ £ £	🪓 🪓🪓 🪓🪓🪓 🪓🪓🪓🪓 🪓🪓🪓🪓🪓	❁ ❁❁ ❁❁❁ ❁❁❁❁ ❁❁❁❁❁	✳ ☁ ☁☁ ☁☁☁ ☁
Where the evidence is uncertain or outcome variable I have tried to indicate this with a query, for example: ❁? or ☁?				

At the end of each section you will see a rating bar with the four symbols to help you decide how easy each approach might be to use.

If an approach is costly; difficult (it would probably require professional help); has a good success rate; but can have significant problems (think of a complicated signature dish you might get in a 5-star restaurant), then you might be able to carry this off at home but only if you were skilled to start with, knew the likely problems and could deal with them.

On the other hand, if the approach is cheap; fairly simple; has a high success rate; and is unlikely to cause any problems (to pursue the cooking analogy, think of this as equivalent to making yourself a cheese sandwich), it should be feasible for most people to try.

I'm sure you get the idea.

An overview of what we know about more general aspects of sleep is given towards the end of the book.

For many people who live every day with ASD, sleep problems come as an unwelcome and unexpected extra. Although common to people with ASD, they are often the 'elephant in the room'. Their effects are significant and wide-ranging, but they can often be missed by professionals or seen as not relevant to the person's ASD. Sometimes, even when they are a significant issue, no clinical help is given.

Other problems are also more common in ASD. Issues affecting the nervous system (including epilepsy and neuromuscular disorders), diabetes and gastrointestinal difficulties are all frequently seen (see, e.g.: Kohane *et al.* 2012). These can also make life more demanding and difficult, and can occur in various combinations. None are as common as sleep disorders, but some of these other issues may be linked to problems with sleep.

Discussion is confined, as far as possible, to the main treatments that might help, and is based on the current best evidence at this time.

Many of these topics were covered in more detail in a book detailing more of the scientific and research background (Aitken 2012). It also discusses a wider range of historical and alternative approaches. I have excluded discussion of many other approaches referred to in reviews, often without proper discussion, or mention of the reasons they have fallen out of favour.

Are sleep problems really all that important?

If I was going to invest my time and effort in trying to sort out a problem, and was offered a treatment for it, I would want to know various things first. How likely is it that the treatment will work, and how much good is it likely to do if it does? I would want to know whether it was really worth my while bothering – could putting in the effort pay off?

Maybe it's just like anything else I could do if I put my mind to it: I could probably learn to whistle the old Persian national anthem if I tried hard enough – I could source CD recordings, practise every night, and with enough time and perseverance I might be able to whistle a passable likeness of it. Somehow I don't think I'll bother even if I could, (a) because it would involve me in a lot of effort and (b) because it isn't going to be of benefit to me.

I strongly believe that sleep problems should be assessed and, where possible, sorted out. Here are some of the reasons (there are many more):

- Children who sleep better perform better at school.

- They develop better planning and problem-solving abilities.

- They have fewer behavioural difficulties like aggression, defiance, non-compliance and self-injury.

- They have better impulse control from preschool through at least into late childhood.

- They have better immune function and lower infection risk.

- Ongoing sleep problems cause distress to everyone in the family.

- Overtired and confused carers are more easily pushed to their own limits.

Finally:

- In adults, severe sleep problems impair quality of life and lead to poorer ability to function at work.

These are not just my views or educated guesswork but summarise a large amount of research.

It's 'official': having poorer sleep can hold back your development, lead you to underachieve and make it harder to notice how your behaviour stresses those around you. It can make you more difficult to spend time with and make it more likely that your parents, partners, brothers, sisters and carers will have a harder time coping with you, and with each other. You are more likely to struggle in many areas – getting and keeping friends, succeeding in your education, keeping in good health and getting and holding down a job.

So, *sleep problems are important.*

But maybe not always. Something that is a problem for everyone else may not be a problem for you. Some children with autism are now being described as having 'contented sleeplessness' and may not need help with sleeping. There is a genuine dilemma here – should we only try help someone to improve their sleep if they are aware of having a difficulty and can tell us that they want to change?

My own view here is that the evidence is strong enough to suggest people with sleep problems should be helped to sleep better even when they are not concerned by it or aware of it as a problem. This will help them develop to the best of their abilities, make them happier and minimise the risk to their physical and mental health.

Poor sleep can cause or worsen mental health issues like anxiety, depression and 'challenging behaviours'. Difficulties with aggression, temper tantrums (or 'meltdowns') and self-injury can be particularly difficult to deal with. They are more commonly seen if there are associated learning problems, but are difficult issues whoever presents with them and irrespective of their ability level.

Problem behaviours are more difficult to control and harder to tolerate when everyone is sleeping more poorly, is overtired and is more likely to get irritated. If your sleep is poor, you can find it harder to understand the world around you – something that is already more difficult for someone with an ASD to do. Parents are more likely to have arguments and fall out with each other, and otherwise minor problems can easily spiral out of control.

Untreated sleep problems can come at enormous cost to the people who have them, to their families and to other carers. Missed days from school or work take their toll on everyone – if you don't get up in time for the school bus and someone has to take time off work to look after you or to take you to school; if your parents have to take time off to accompany you to clinic appointments; if your brothers and sisters can't practise, revise or study because they are overtired… I am sure these issues and many others will be only too familiar to many people reading this.

The financial impact on families can be significant when people have to take unpaid time off work or are unable to do overtime because they are too tired. It can be hard to explain to your employer that your work is suffering because someone else has a sleep problem but the issue can be all too real.

In addition to the strain on families, the wider economic cost of sleep problems can be truly staggering. One study found that lost productivity from adult insomnia in Quebec alone amounted to £3.2 billion every year (Daley *et al.* 2009).

Some general issues

You may think that this next section is just common sense, but I hope that you don't skip over it. Try to take the time to read it next. Sometimes the obvious really is what works best, but often what seems common sense turns out to be wrong. Many popular sayings have opposites: 'Many hands make light work' and 'Too many cooks spoil the broth' come to mind as examples. Both can be right, but not usually at the same time.

How can you try to disentangle truth from hearsay (see: Watts 2011)? This is something that needs a bit of time and effort – there are no magic wands.

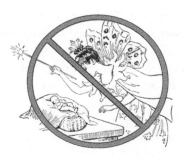

No magic wands

How dwelling on the past can get you stuck with problems in the present

Severe sleep problems you can't understand are often more exhausting than similar issues you half expected and feel you do.

Many approaches begin with taking a detailed background history and trying to understand how it started. This assumes that understanding what started it will help to sort it. Everything has a history, and seeing why a problem might have arisen feels right. This could help you to understand it and might make it easier to tolerate it and to see a solution.

But knowing how something began often doesn't help sort it. Why?

Let's use a different example: your car runs out of fuel on a deserted road at night. You could get a detailed history, including checking the last time you filled the tank, your mileage since then and how you have been driving. This might help explain why you ran dry. Other details – how you were feeling about your car at the time, whether you had considered trading it in recently and whether you had neglected to book its last service on time – may be easy to collect but largely irrelevant to the problem.

No matter how good the history, and your understanding of the problem, only refuelling is likely to sort the problem – this is what you need now, not to understand how the problem arose.

Conclusions about the past are almost always educated guesswork. We can't be absolutely sure that the things we focus on, or recall, were really the important factors. All of us have selective recall and will remember things differently for a host of reasons (this is just as true in other areas – 'We always knew something was wrong', 'She was fine until she got…').

We can't change the past. Without breaking the laws of physics, the past is going to stay there and won't change no matter how well we understand the consequences or what we do about it. Knowing about it might help us to avoid similar things happening again but will not be likely to sort the problem you are having now.

Let's take a sleep example:

▬ Logan is 15. He has recurring nightmares when he clearly imagines being attacked by a group of boys in a back alley and getting badly kicked and bruised. Not long before they began, he had been the victim of a real-life gang attack in a dark alleyway that had left him badly bruised and shaken. Afterwards it had been difficult for him to sleep because he was really uncomfortable whenever he lay down. The physical aches gradually subsided but his difficulties with sleeping have persisted. They interfere with his school work, and he is reluctant to go out.

Logan's doctor has referred him to a psychotherapist for help. He has reassured him that nightmares are normal after such trauma. He told Logan, 'Obviously you will have unresolved issues around the assault and in your nightmares you seem to replay the attack again and again. This is quite normal and will gradually resolve over time. Don't worry about them.'

Logan gets on well with his therapist, he understands the explanation and is relieved to know that he is responding normally. He also avoids situations where he might get attacked again. What he really wants is therapy to stop his nightmares rather than a better understanding of why they are still happening. He still wakes screaming at 2am feeling terrified, often waking everyone else. He doesn't want this to keep happening to him. He wants it to stop, not just to understand it better.

Most of us will have had some dreams or nightmares that we remember. Often what we remember overlaps with memories of real events. I had vivid dreams around the time of the finals for my first degree. In the dreams I was studying for my exams and I started to worry that I might confuse things I dreamed with the real things I had learned for the exams.

Investigating what happened around the time someone's nightmares started can often point to things that help explain them. The difficulty with this approach to interpreting the content of dreams as the focus of therapy is that by identifying historical events it emphasises things we can't change and gives us a reason our problems are likely to continue.

It is better to concentrate on current sleep behaviour, looking at what you might be able to change rather than explaining why things might have happened or why people think particular approaches might help.

Unlike past events, what is happening now is changeable. It makes more sense to try to keep focused on things that you can change rather than historical reasons for the problem.

But, just as with past problems, with current ones there are loads of possible reasons why there is a sleep problem here and now.

If you have found a plausible reason why the problem may have started off, you may want to see if this is still an issue.

In order to find the best approach to sorting out any difficulty, you need a clear idea what is maintaining it.

Why there isn't one simple solution to sleep problems

It is tempting to look at a solution someone else has found to be effective and just try doing what they did. If you do, you might be lucky and get similar results, but remember that the same factors don't always apply, and one approach does not help with all problems, so no treatment is a 'one size fits all' solution.

This is one reason so many people are disappointed that they don't suddenly look like a film star/lose masses of weight/become sexually irresistible when they try the latest 'sure-fire' approach they read about. It might have worked for the person you saw being interviewed on the programme, but everyone is different (even identical twins) and these individual differences are often critically important.

As we will see, there are many different types of sleep problem and many possible approaches; some work well with some problems and not with others. Nothing is guaranteed to work with everyone – as someone once said, the only certainties in life are death and taxes.

'You get what you wish for'
(how your beliefs can affect what happens)

■— **Take 1:** Sam felt he was in poor physical shape and decided to do something about it. He saw a personal fitness instructor who assessed him and put him on an exercise and diet regime based on these results to help him slim down, build up his strength and improve his muscle tone. However successful this turns out to be, Sam's aim is to get in better shape. Both Sam and the instructor now believe that his fitness level can be improved – Sam wants to get himself in better shape, and aim to start from his current ability level.

So Sam believes: I can get myself in better shape, I know how to do it. I just need to get cracking!

This seems common sense. Many people who are concerned about their health change their diet and go on an exercise regime. There is a massive industry catering to our obsessions with fitness, weight control and body shape, and the equipment, clothing, exercise spaces and nutrition to help us. Much of this provides unrealistic goals, poorly thought out ideas and bad advice (an excellent overview can be found in Taubes 2007), but many people do manage to lose weight, get fitter and more toned and some manage to keep it up.

▬ **Take 2:** Sam felt he was in poor physical shape and decided to do something about it. He saw a lifestyle coach who took his family history and arranged for some genetic tests. It seemed that his poor physical condition was inevitable and unchangeable – he had a genetic profile that made him more likely to gain weight and his father and uncle had both put on excess weight when they were around Sam's age. Sam accepted that his poor physical shape was a consequence of his lifestyle and his genetic make-up. He has concluded there is nothing that he can do to alter his fitness level or to combat his ever-expanding waistline. He feels he has been dealt a bad hand by his biology and that there is nothing he can do to alter the inevitable.

So Sam believes: Nothing I do is likely to alter my chances of gaining weight – it's genetically predetermined, I just have bad Kismet, so why bother?

This second scenario is not too far-fetched either. One hundred and thirty separate genes have been found linked to an increased risk of becoming overweight (Jiménez 2011). Obesity does tend to run in families. A number of private companies now offer individualised genetic profiling, and off-the-shelf risk profiling for specific problems will be available soon. We probably all know people who have had their weight gain put down to 'slow metabolism' and just accepted this as inevitable.

Of course there is logic and some truth at both extremes. If Sam trained regularly at his ideal tolerance level, ate an optimal diet, slept well and enhanced his performance by training with the best advice and equipment he could afford, he would be disappointed and incredibly unlucky if his general fitness and performance at his chosen sport did not improve but, equally, given his age and track record so far, he has no realistic chance of being in a medal position at the next Olympics however much he tries.

> **So Sam believes:** I can get slimmer and fitter, take up sports I didn't consider previously, improve my health, my social life and my life expectancy but I accept there are limits and I will never become a 'perfect' specimen.

It is easy to think yourself into a position where you seem unable to do anything to sort out a problem because it feels as if you are at the mercy of inevitability. If you believe you can't alter things, you have talked yourself into accepting the problem. If you can focus on the here and now and what is maintaining it, you can start to see if change is a realistic goal.

At the opposite extreme is believing that nothing is beyond you. If you start to believe that nothing is impossible, and you can become the slimmest/strongest/fittest/fastest, your inability to measure up is going to cause problems. Pretty soon you will be disillusioned by your own failure to make progress: 'Look at me, I can't even benchpress 700kg/do 1000 step-ups without a break/run a three-minute-mile/beat my last marathon time...'

Sleep problems are no different – if you have a significant problem, you should be able to sleep better than you have been doing, and although you may not end up with the best sleeping pattern in the world, you would be incredibly unlucky if you couldn't improve your sleep. Studying and making use of the advice given in this book should help you to be realistic about what can be achieved and increase your chances of achieving it.

So, if you want to try to sort things out what do you need to do next?

1. **Collect information to help define the problem:** Probably starting with a 'baseline' record of the night-to-night pattern you hope to change.

2. **Identify what it is:** From the information you gather, see if you can clarify the sort of sleep difficulty you are dealing with.

Once you have done this:

3. **Try to find an approach that could work:** See if there is an approach that is feasible and has a reasonable chance of helping.

Try to figure out what you can change and what you can't

Most adults have a whole host of failed ambitions. These are usually things you wanted to achieve or avoid. It is no surprise that few people make a resolution to keep things just as they are. 'I want to be like that, I don't want to be like this.' Start by recognising that it is often hard to achieve and maintain change.

Understanding why something keeps happening is the first step towards managing it. This idea may seem strange, but it is far more important to identify what is maintaining a problem (something that you might be able to change) than trying to figure out why it might have started (something that you will never be sure of and are never going to alter). You can change many things that are continuing to happen, but not the past. If you have been obsessed with historical questions – 'Where did we go wrong?', 'What have we done?' 'What didn't we do?'– it is time to move on and refocus. What is happening that you can change?

Those with ASD aren't the only people who sleep poorly – it is how bad the problem is and how long it tends to last that are different, not the sorts of sleep difficulties. Many of the approaches that work for others with sleep difficulties can work equally well.

Sometimes, however, as we go on to see, there are real biological differences that disturb sleep in the ASDs. These tend to make the problems more obvious rather than making them totally different. Although tried and tested methods can often help, it would be naive to say that everyone with ASD who has a sleep problem responds as expected.

For some people's problems there are, as yet, no proven and effective approaches. This does not mean that nothing is going to help. It may be just that no research has so far been done on effective methods. An 'absence of evidence' (the lack of research into what could work) is not the same as having 'evidence of absence' (good research showing that nothing helps).

There is an unfortunate tendency for professionals to do nothing if published evidence is lacking, justifying inaction on the basis of a lack of adequate evidence. Often there isn't a good enough level of published evidence for recommended best practice to have emerged. Even if we put to one side the lack of good comparative evidence for most approaches, there is a need for greater emphasis on how to help.

I am not recommending that you try anything if there is no recommended conventional approach. A good 'single-case' method should be used to assess a plausible and safe intervention (whatever this might be). You need to collect evidence on the problem and on whether what you do works.

It is also important to know whether there is research that shows what is ineffective or best avoided, especially where there can be harmful side-effects. In the past there may have been repeated attempts to treat similar problems with a specific approach to no benefit and it is wasting time to repeat things that don't work.

Understand when you might be able to tackle things
by yourself and when you might need some help
Most sleep issues can be tackled with techniques that families should be able to carry out for themselves once they have the idea – improving sleep hygiene and the majority of behavioural approaches can be used by families without much need for further advice or guidance. Where prescription medication is needed, or biomedical assessments have to be carried out and interpreted, the involvement of a clinician with the requisite skills is required. Some approaches like cognitive-behavioural therapies are likely to be more effective when implemented by a trained therapist.

You shouldn't try to carry out an approach you don't understand or one that is difficult to implement without any support.

PART A

YOU THINK THERE IS A PROBLEM, SO WHAT CAN YOU DO ABOUT IT?

A flock of sheep that leisurely pass by
One after one; the sound of rain, and bees
Murmuring; the fall of rivers, winds and seas,
Smooth fields, white sheets of water, and pure sky –
I've thought of all by turns, and still I lie
Sleepless...

(William Wordsworth, 'To Sleep')

— 1 —

SLEEP PROBLEMS

Imagine you have booked your car for a service. The mechanics need to know the make, model, year it was made, any changes or refinements it has had, date of its last service and any problems you've been having with it. This helps them know if it might need new spark plugs/an oil change/aircon recharge/wheel realignment/they might need to order specific parts/use non-metric tools…

With a popular make and model of car, experienced mechanics can tell what they may need and will have appropriate experience.

Whatever the car, a number of things will be done during a routine service – oil change, brake fluid, filters, etc., but even these will differ for some models. Even the best local mechanics will probably need to do some homework if you happen to have an unusual vehicle.

Let's assume that you have read this far because the obvious things you have tried haven't worked. You need to think about difficult sleep problems like the mechanic – some things are fairly standard so it's easy to say what to do, others may be very different and might require you to do some homework. If you can look at the problem this way it should help you to find what can work.

— 2 —

WHAT SORTS OF SLEEP PROBLEMS ARE THERE?

Two main systems define and classify sleep problems – let's call these 'workshop manuals' to keep with the car analogy. The International Classification of Sleep Disorders-2 (ICSD-2) (American Academy of Sleep Medicine 2005) describes eight main types of sleeping difficulties as well as night-time wetting and night-time soiling. The Diagnostic and Statistical Manual of the American Psychiatric Association (usually shortened to 'DSM') in its latest version, DSM-5, introduced in May 2013, classifies 14 specific sleep problems (American Psychiatric Association 2013). Already you can see that the number of possible 'models' differs depending on the classification you use.

Table A1 compares the two classifications, and also gives some other terms clinicians might use. Don't be put off by complicated-sounding words. These are just labels that help you to be clearer about what you are dealing with. If you need to remind yourself what a particular term stands for, there is a glossary at the back of this book with short descriptions.

Not every possible sleep disorder or night-time problem is covered under ICSD-2 or DSM-5. 'New' problems are regularly being described. For example, 'night-time eating disorders' have only recently made an appearance in the sleep literature.

Next you need to get a good description of your problem – this is like identifying the model and creating your own DIY service manual.

Table A1: Sleep problem classification

The ICSD-2 system	The DSM-5 system	Reported sleep problem/disorder
American Academy of Sleep Medicine (2005)	American Psychiatric Association (2013)	Other terms that might be used to describe general sleep problems
Insomnia	Primary insomnia Insomnia Insomnia + substance abuse Insomnia + sleep efficiency comorbid mental health disorder	Settling difficulties Co-sleeping issues Night-waking Long sleep latency Early waking Difficult bedtime routines Daytime sleepiness
Parasomnias	Parasomnia disorders	Nightmares Awakening screaming Nocturnal enuresis
Hypersomnias of central origin	Kleine-Levin syndrome Primary hypersomnia	Kleine-Levin syndrome Hypersomnia Daytime sleepiness
Sleep-related breathing disorders	Obstructive sleep apnoea-hypopnoea syndrome Primary central sleep apnoea Primary alveolar hypoventilation	Obstructive sleep apnoea
Sleep-related movement disorders	Restless legs syndrome	Periodic limb movements in sleep (PLMS) Restless sleep

Circadian rhythm sleep disorders	Circadian rhythm sleep disorder
	  Delayed sleep phase type
	  Jet lag type
	  Shift work type
	  Free-running type
	  Irregular sleep–wake type
	(All of the above are subsumed under the new category of narcolepsy-cataplexy)
		Late sleep onset
		Long sleep latency
		Irregular sleep–wake patterns
		Free-running sleep

Isolated symptoms	–	Short sleep/hyposomnia Early waking
Other sleep disorders	–	Abnormal objective sleep patterns (on actigraphy)

― 3 ―

HOW COMMON ARE DIFFERENT SLEEP PROBLEMS?

Mild sleep problems affect around a quarter of all children. Some specific issues are even more common. Snoring happens nightly in around one in ten people, but few are identified or treated. Sleep problems are more common in clinical groups like ASD, ADHD (attention-deficit hyperactivity disorder) and with growth problems.

Sleep issues are consistently reported to be common in children and adolescents and often lead to other problems if not identified and treated. Fortunately, the same approaches seem to help, whether or not there are any other difficulties (Harvey *et al.* 2010). Many childhood sleep problems, however, go undiagnosed and ignored (Blunden *et al.* 2004).

— 4 —

HOW YOU CAN WORK
OUT WHAT MIGHT HELP

*...recognize out of a number of facts which are incidental
and which vital. Otherwise your energy and attention
must be dissipated instead of being concentrated.*

(Sherlock Holmes, in *The Reigate Squires*,
Arthur Conan Doyle, 1893)

Being 'a bit of a Sherlock Holmes' –
the art and science of problem-solving

With a sleep problem, you want to find a reliable and safe approach
with a good chance of helping. You need to start by figuring out the
clues in your latest case.

So, let's get detecting. What do you already know and what do
you need to find out?

- What evidence do you already have?

- What new evidence might you need?

- Has anyone published research on similar cases?

- What can you rule out (it can sometimes be just as important
  to know what something isn't as what it is)?

- What has and hasn't worked in earlier cases that seem similar?

And, by combining the above:

- What approach might have a reasonable chance of helping?

Some cases can be solved at home – most sleep problems are sorted without any input from professionals – but for various reasons others might require outside help:

- A particular approach may be too difficult or too tiring to implement without help (for example, 'dry bed training' is far easier if you have the help of people who are used to being awake through the night, than if you have to stay up for several nights yourself while still trying to hold down a day job).

- Some approaches may require a prescription medication or supplements.

- You may need more specialised medical input if the person has other difficulties like asthma, seizures, anxiety problems, ADHD or a heart condition (all of which are also more common in someone with ASD).

- The sleep problem may be part of a more complicated picture (there may be additional problems like parental depression or other family issues).

- Assessment may need specialised equipment (such as overnight sleep recording).

When the evidence suggests an approach is effective with the particular type of sleep problem you have identified, you have a strategy. If you implement it and the problem improves, you have 'solved' your first case!

Things may turn out to be more complicated and you might need to involve a professional. An experienced clinician may be better placed to decipher the clues and work out the best approach. No matter, by then you should have done a lot of the groundwork – getting your baseline and ruling out more obvious possibilities and the next stage should be faster and easier.

The next sections tell you how to build a clearer idea of the sleep issue you are dealing with and how to collect the information you will need.

So, what is the problem you need to try to sort?

Before you can go on to look through possible treatments and decide what is relevant, you need to try to be clear about what the problem is. Unless you know the name of the problem, for example, you can't search for what's been tried previously, or search for new treatments.

1. First, gather evidence about the problem – get a 'baseline'.

2. Once you have your evidence, see how well you can describe and define the problem – does this give you clues that are good enough to be specific about what the problem is?

3. How does it compare to previous cases? (Hardly anyone presents with a truly unique type of sleep difficulty, but no two problems will be identical.)

4. What has worked for others?

5. Is there a successful approach you think you could use?

If you have a clear idea of an approach to try:

6. Plan how to carry it out.

7. Decide if you will need help.

And:

8. Having done all of this, try to record changes. Why this is important:

   ○ It tells you if it is working.

   ○ It helps you to 'fine-tune' things.

   ○ You can remember what helped if the problem returns.

   ○ You will have 'proof' if you need to show anyone else.

(Families often have difficulty convincing agencies about earlier success. This applies to all sorts of interventions, not just with sleep – without good recording it is just a matter of whether you are believed. If you have written dated records this can make things much easier.)

Take a minute to run through the 'sleep checklist' in Box A1. If you can identify one or more possible issues, you might want to read the section at the beginning of Section B now and then come back to this part.

BOX A1: SLEEP CHECKLIST

- Is the problem with getting to sleep at night?
- Do they wake very early and have problems getting back to sleep?
- Do they sleep or get excessively tired during the day?
- Do they wake up in distress?
- Do they sleepwalk or talk in their sleep?
- Do they ever wet or dirty themselves when asleep?
- Do they snore?
- Do they sleep for longer than normal?
- Are they overweight?
- Have they had or have they been suspected of having epilepsy?
- Do they get recurrent ear infections?
- Do they have good dental health?

You will need clear information about how bad the problem is. All parents and carers worry about their children – this is perfectly normal. Can you be sure that you are concerned because there is a significant problem or could you be worrying unduly as many parents do?

— 5 —

FINDING OUT ABOUT
YOUR PROBLEM

Starting to keep a record

Your first step is usually to *keep a diary of the pattern.* This gives you
something to compare against (a suggested diary outline is provided
in Appendix 5). You may need to record some things that are fairly
specific, so a general one-size-fits-all diary isn't always going to be
good enough – check the next section for ideas of what you might
want to record and start making a list.

Ideally, record for long enough that you can see a clear pattern. If
there are only problems on a couple of nights each week this might
take a couple of weeks for you to do; if the night-to-night pattern is
familiar and much the same then keeping a diary for a week might
be enough; if the problem is infrequent – say you are worried about
severe nightmares that only happen every few weeks, you might need
to record for longer.

You are probably the best judge of what is typical and of whether
your diary shows the usual pattern.

(I remember working with a boy a few years ago who was referred
with a phobia about thunder and lightning. We used an elaborate set-
up with sound archive thunder recordings and borrowed photographic
flashlights to simulate a storm – this was surprisingly realistic when
we had him lying back with his eyes shut. Initially this provoked a
severe phobic response, but after a few sessions he could lie through
a simulated thunderstorm without becoming distressed. Case closed –
he felt better, and could go out if it looked like rain when he had been
housebound before. We had to wait months for a storm to brew up
before we could be sure that the treatment worked to help him cope
with real thunder and lightning.)

If you think, 'This feels too much like schoolwork, maybe I'll just skip it'

Try to remember that, without keeping a record, it can be difficult to know whether there really is a problem. However tempting, try not to plough on regardless without collecting this sort of evidence as you go. If you put things in place to correct a real problem but haven't documented it first, it can be difficult to show improvement. It will be difficult to convince anyone else that what you did made a difference; if the problem recurs it can make it harder to remember what worked or how long it took. A diary record helps you remember the pattern, what changed, and is a good starting point for anyone else needing to understand the problem.

Looking through your evidence

> *It is an old maxim of mine that when you have*
> *excluded the impossible, whatever remains,*
> *however improbable, must be the truth.*

> (Sherlock Holmes, in *The Adventure of the Beryl Coronet*, Arthur Conan Doyle, 1892)

Once you have your diary and have collected any other relevant evidence, look for patterns that might help you decide what to do next – clinicians sometimes call this a 'functional analysis'. Don't make assumptions about what the problem will be – see what evidence you have, and whether it suggests a pattern.

Trying to understand the problem

You need a way of sifting through your clues. This is something you will need to do in some form whatever approach you decide on.

Can you see any pattern in the sleep diary? It helps to have a structure. One thing that can often help is to look for differences that might give you a lead. Often it helps if there are some nights/times that the problem doesn't occur. Maybe it never happens at weekends or on holidays, or when someone is staying over.

Usually you need to look at three things:

1. What leads up to it (the **A**ntecedents).

2. What the problem is (the **B**ehaviour itself).

3. What happens after (its **C**onsequences).

This is sometimes called an ABC approach. It helps to identify the problem, and any related issues (see Table A2).

Table A2: The ABC approach

	A Antecedents (what leads up to it)	B Behaviour (what the problem is)	C Consequences (what happens after)
Setting events	Problems during day? Time getting to bed? Activities before bed? Bath/shower? Supper?	Who is there? Where is it? What time is it? Is there a reason?	Do they disturb anyone? Does anyone else react? Does anyone have to go to see to them? Do they settle?
Behaviour	Upsets Arguments Excitement Fighting Being bullied Anticipation of problem	Frequency Intensity Number within episode Duration	Do they wake? Do they get up?

Two other sorts of information can help. The first is a description of the situation the problem happens in (often called its 'setting events'). The second is a description of what the problem is (its 'parameters').

Finding out what else is going on

A good way to remember this one is to think of the 'five Ws' – **W**ho? **W**hat? **W**here? **W**hen? and **W**hy? These are the *setting events* in which the problem happens.

*   ***Who* is present when it happens?** Do they share a bed or room? Do they fall asleep elsewhere and get carried to bed? Does someone stay with them until they fall asleep? Who sees to them if they waken and need to be settled?

- *What* **do they do?** Is the pattern always the same or does it vary? If it varies, is this systematic? (e.g. do they cause more of an issue if settled to bed by a specific person or only relate well to one carer?)

- *Where* **does it happen?** Do they always sleep in the same bed/place? What happens on holidays/when in hospital/at relatives or friends?

- *When* **does it happen?** This is where a sleep diary can help a lot – is the pattern consistent or is there a particular pattern to the variability? (e.g. more broken nights after a good unbroken night/bedwetting/a nocturnal seizure? Is it better at weekends or on weekdays? Is it linked to any other events – variation in bedtime; family arguments…?) If the problem is long-standing, does it differ at different times of the year?

  In girls, if they have started their periods, is there any link to the menstrual cycle? Remember that this could be in the person with the sleep issue, but could also be an issue relating to a mother, sister or carer.

- *Why* **does it happen?** Does anything in the patterns that emerge from the above suggest what might be maintaining the problem?

Describing the sleep problem

People often use the term 'FINDS' to help them remember what to look at here. This stands for the **F**requency, **I**ntensity, **N**umber, **D**uration and **S**ense of the things that are happening. These are a way of describing what someone does and can be used to indicate how severe it is.

- **Frequency:** How often do they do 'it' (e.g. waking; screaming; wetting) – every night/week/month?

- **Intensity:** How extreme is it when it occurs? (If they wake up, do they become roused but fall back to sleep quietly/wake and sit up in bed/become fully awake and get out of bed/ need someone to settle them…?)

- **Number:** How often does the problem occur on a typical night? (e.g. if they wake up with a nightmare, is this several times a night; once a night; most nights; once every few nights; about once a week; sporadically; only on school nights; only at weekends...?)

- **Duration:** How long does each episode last for (hours/ minutes/fleetingly)?

- **Sense:** Does there seem to be anything obvious that might be maintaining the problem (they get to go into parents' bed/their own bedroom is cold/there is a lot of street noise/wind...)?

You may be starting to see a pattern. For example, you might identify something outside the home that you hadn't expected and that other people aren't disturbed by, like noise from people returning home from a new bar with a late licence that has opened locally; the motor kicking in on the refrigerator late at night; the new neighbour's cats fighting on the lawn...

If the problem has only become a recent concern, did anything else change around the same time?

It could become obvious that something you have not recorded seems to relate to the problem — let's say that you notice that night terrors seem to have happened mainly on the nights when another child was arguing with you over their homework. You may want to record for a bit longer to see if this seems really important, adding this new issue in to your records.

Finding a pattern

We are looking for a way to sort through clues and see a pattern. I have presented this as a diagram (Figure A1) that can help you to recognise how issues might interrelate (see: Morton 2004 for an early version of this way of looking at patterns in behaviour).

Let's see how you might use it. There are four headings: biology; cognition; behaviour; and consequences. You could include any other issues/information that seem relevant — relationships (issues such as separation anxiety); emotional content/reactions (of nightmares or worrying dreams); family reactions (to behaviours like sleepwalking or bedwetting); or events outside the home (like being bullied in school affecting anxiety), as required.

Paul is a 9-year-old 'high-functioning' autistic boy, who has been referred for help with his sleep. He has a history of insomnia. His diet is very self-restricted, he gets extremely worried about any situations where he is asked to join in with others, and his school are concerned that he is underachieving. His family were given some initial sleep advice from a support group and now have a regular night-time routine in place.

He has been put through a battery of physical tests. These showed that he has a low level of acetylserotonin methyltransferase (ASMT) activity. Genetic screening found a deletion on his Y chromosome in the coding region for this enzyme (Yp11.32).

The lower level of enzyme activity means that Paul makes less melatonin than normal. His salivary melatonin has been assessed and is roughly half the normal age-expected level for a boy of 9. On the plus side, it showed a normal circadian pattern, with higher levels in early evening and lowest levels around lunchtime. An assessment by a dietician found that his self-restricted diet is low in tryptophan, an essential dietary precursor to melatonin.

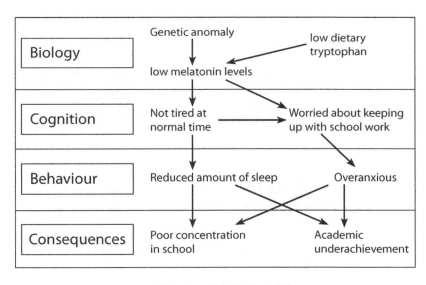

Figure A1: The CDU model

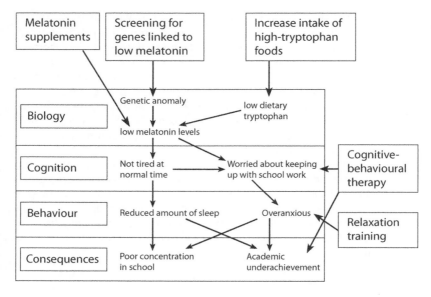

Figure A2: A worked example of the CDU model

Using the model, various relevant issues can be identified (Figure A2). Any of these could be important to Paul's case as I have described it and several or all of them might have to be changed before his sleep improves.

The following seem the most likely factors to be relevant to helping Paul:

1. Paul's low melatonin levels suggest that melatonin supplements might be helpful in increasing his sleep, reducing anxiety and improving his academic performance.

2. Counselling about the genetic finding could help make sense of the problem for Paul and his family and help other affected family members to understand and manage their own difficulties.

3. Paul might benefit from increasing his intake of high-tryptophan foods (see: Aitken 2008). His genetic difference makes it less likely that this will help. He has a circadian pattern of melatonin release and the earlier steps in this pathway that alter tryptophan to make acetylserotonin seem to be working normally.

4. Cognitive-behavioural therapy could help Paul to deal with his anxiety and improve his academic performance (see: Wood *et al.* 2006).

5. Relaxation training might provide Paul with a method to control his anxiety and is a practical strategy to use at bedtime.

This example should help people to see how various strands can affect a sleep issue and why good problem-solving may suggest new possibilities.

Why it can be so difficult to do what would work

Sleep problems are often part of more general family difficulties. When you are in the middle of a difficult situation it can be hard to see what is going on and how you are reacting to it – you just do the best you can.

This is something called a 'coercive family process', a pattern seen in many long-standing difficult behaviours. When this develops, no one involved enjoys it but everyone is rewarded, in some sense, and feels they are dealing with things as best they can. Recognising the pattern can be a major step in starting to sort things out.

Let's use an example to highlight a coercive pattern:

— Ellie has a problem with her 3-year-old daughter Susie. More specifically, she is infuriated with Susie's constant interruptions whenever she is on the phone.

From the outside we can see that Susie has developed a cunning and successful plan. Let's call it: 'Susie's "Getting Mum off the phone so she can play with me" plan.'

Susie is very close to her mother. Every time Ellie is on the phone to a friend at home for more than a few minutes, Susie gets bored and annoyed and starts to shout. She keeps herself out of Ellie's reach and always makes enough noise so that Ellie has to finish her call in order to settle her. Usually Ellie is annoyed and tells her off. The telling off gets Susie upset, and neither of them really enjoys what is happening. Ellie often ends up consoling Susie and feeling guilty.

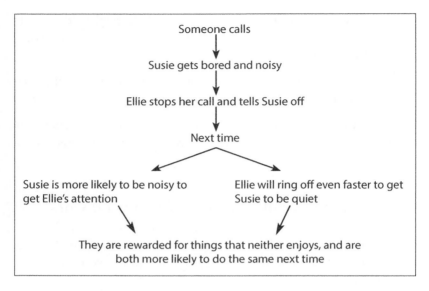

Figure A3: The coercive family process

Susie has worked out how to get Ellie's attention when she is on the phone, and Ellie has worked out how to get Susie to be quiet – they both get a pay-off for their behaviour. Neither is really achieving what they want and neither enjoys the process.

When you start to see the pattern, it gets easier to change it. In this example, Ellie could use various strategies to help her ignore Susie. This is the difficult bit for Ellie – she always feels guilty afterwards and wonders if she gives Susie enough of her time, but also worries that all the time she spends calming Susie and cutting her friends' calls short is losing her some of her best friends.

What could Ellie do?

There are lots of possibilities:

- Arrange with friends to chat on the phone when Susie is asleep so the problem doesn't occur. This is feasible but does not teach Susie about being quiet when Mum is on the phone.

- Pretend to call someone and just have a one-sided conversation with herself while holding the phone to her ear.

- Prepare a friend beforehand, call her, and ignore Susie's disruptive behaviour while talking and keeping going until Susie quietens (Figure A4).

Doing any of these could make it easier for Ellie to practise ignoring Susie being noisy, and allow her to reward Susie for being quiet instead.

- Ellie could install an answerphone – this would reduce the number of incidents but doesn't really address the problem, which is Susie's behaviour when Ellie takes a call.

Susie needs to learn what is acceptable when Mum is on the phone so they can both get something positive from these times.

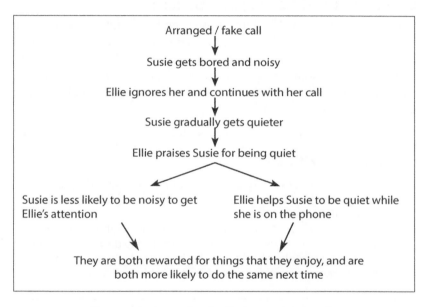

Figure A4: A coercive family process intervention

Once Ellie saw the problem, she could see why she was finding it so difficult. She had a short-term strategy for dealing with Susie but hadn't realised it rewarded Susie by giving her attention when she was doing exactly what Ellie wanted her to stop. No wonder it wasn't getting any better. Once she saw the problem and also what she could do to change things, it boosted her confidence – she *could* understand her daughter after all! It helped Susie by giving her the attention she wanted without being so disruptive and made her time with her mum more fun.

This model can be widely applied to many family-based behavioural problems (see: Paterson 1982).

It should be fairly easy to see how the pattern can be a part of some sleep problems. With settling problems and frequent night-waking, the child may get comforted or one-to-one attention. The same can be true of more difficult or distressing behaviours like soiling, wetting or night-time self-injury. As with Susie's shouting, seeing the pattern gives a better understanding and an idea of how to change it.

What if you have described and studied the problem but still can't see a pattern?

Some sleep issues in ASD are unusual and difficult to understand. They might have a physical basis and require assessments that can't be carried out easily without access to hospital facilities. Sometimes videosomnography is the most revealing (this is where an electroencephalograph (EEG) and video are recorded simultaneously while the person is asleep).

IN A NUTSHELL

Before you try to tackle a problem *it helps to know what the problem is and how bad it is*. This makes it easier to tell if anything you do is making a difference.

In this section we have discussed and described the importance of getting the right information together to help you decide what your problem is; how to identify basic issues; how to tell whether problem-solving strategies are working, and how to check on your progress.

Next, you need to make sure you have the basics in place to minimise night-time arousal and disruption, and create a good bedtime routine.

— 6 —

WAYS TO SORT OUT
SLEEP PROBLEMS

Knowing is not enough; we must apply.
Willing is not enough, we must do.

(Johann Wolfgang von Goethe,
1749–1832, German Polymath)

Doing a basic sleep clean-up

A ruffled mind makes a restless pillow.

(Charlotte Brontë, *The Professor*, 1857)

Heightened senses

Some years ago I did a sponsored cycle from Scotland to Bavaria, travelling light and camping out. I remember stopping late one evening in Saarbrücken, an industrial town in the Ruhr valley, and pitching my tent in a small site on the edge of the university playing fields. This was the only time I can ever remember being woken up by smell alone. I discovered the next morning that the campsite was next to some sort of chemical works. There was obviously an industrial process that periodically released something into the air with a truly noxious smell. So much for my camping trip to Bavaria.

People with ASD often have heightened senses, and this can be for taste, touch, sight, sound or smell.

'Hyperacusis' or acute hearing is common, and can sometimes make background noise difficult to tolerate. I had one patient who lived in a semi-detached cottage and whose bedroom adjoined her neighbour's kitchen. She found the noise from the next-door fridge impossible to sleep through. The problem was sorted easily by sleeping in a different room.

'Hyperosmia' or heightened sense of smell is also common. I remember working with one girl who had Asperger syndrome and was in mainstream school. She had extreme tactile sensitivity which made dressing and undressing very difficult. At one point, she became very distressed by the smell of burning from a warehouse fire that happened opposite her school. She commented on being distracted by the smell from this fire for weeks after the event, when her classmates were only aware of it for the first couple of days after the fire.

If someone has heightened sensory awareness it may contribute to sleep difficulties and it may help to have an assessment like the Dunn Sensory Profile carried out (Dunn 1999). This is typically carried out by an occupational therapist (OT), but not all OTs are trained in this.

The sensory environment

Our senses are complex, subtle, and can be difficult to define or describe. We can be sensitive to wide ranges of different factors; many are enjoyable but others may confuse, disorient, frighten or distress.

Edinburgh, where I grew up, is steeped in history, rich in cultures and cuisines and in sensations that intrigue the nostrils. For many years it was a brewing and distilling centre – the smells of roasting grain and fermenting hops were a constant feature.

At one time I worked within 'smelling distance' of the city's slaughterhouse. The complex smells this produced, readily associated with death, were uncomfortable, easy to place, and must have been similar to the smells of carnage in human battlefields of old.

Today, the smell of fresh bread being baked is common in the early hours of an Edinburgh morning, and the cosmopolitan aromas from Asian and Chinese cooking and freshly brewed coffee linger enticingly around many parts of the town, particularly in the early evening. All evoke pleasant memories and are part of the make-up of my sense of Edinburgh. I can imagine, though, that if any of these were distressing to me and my sense of smell was more acute, some might evoke something like the distressed and fitful sleep that I remember on my night's camping in Saarbrücken.

With a sleep problem, there could be something particular to the environment that is more of an issue than normal. In addition to assessing the person, an assessment of where they sleep could also be useful. Initially this might be seeing whether anyone else has difficulty sleeping in the same room and noting if there are situations where the sleep problems don't arise. Do they sleep soundly when at a relative's or when on school trips or on holiday? These might give you clues about what is different about situations where the person sleeps well.

Occasionally some factor, obvious once it is identified, could be having a major effect on sleep. In one case I remember working with, a young girl who lived in a high-rise apartment block was referred with the sudden onset of sleep difficulties in early January. She would come running through to her parents' room late at night in distress. It didn't take long to work out that her bedroom was directly below a boy whose parents had bought him a drum kit as a Christmas present. He was practising at night, loudly but without much ability, with his new present.

All that may be needed is improved 'sleep hygiene'. Sleep hygiene covers a number of aspects of the daily routine and environment that affect sleep. If these changes sort the problem, then a more specific 'problem-focused' approach may not be needed.

There are a few basic sleep hygiene 'rules':

For children

- Try to discourage them from playing on/in their bed in the evening.

- Try to encourage them to associate being in bed with being calm and with sleeping.

- Have a clear pre-agreed bedtime that you remind them about.

- Have a regular bedtime routine – washing, brushing teeth, getting into nightclothes.

- Wind down in the 40 minutes before going to bed – no laptops, computer games, texting, radio, TV or music.

- Try to have a calm pre-sleep activity like a bedtime story/ reading time/story tape that they enjoy and select.

- Keep the lighting level low or lights off in the bedroom.

- Darken the bedroom at bedtime.

For adolescents

- Encourage them to avoid using bed/bedroom for activities other than sleeping.

- Encourage them to prepare for bed when starting to feel tired.

- Try to avoid tobacco in the hours leading up to bedtime.

- Limit coffee, tea and stimulant drinks in the two hours before bed.

- Avoid heavy exercise before bed.

- Wind down in the 40 minutes before going to bed – avoid using laptops, computer games, texting, watching TV or listening to radio or music.

- Keep the lighting low or off in the bedroom.

- Darken the bedroom at bedtime.

Improving sleep hygiene can improve sleep (see: Mindell *et al.* 2009). When things like electronic gadgets (Internet, texting, mobile phones, DVD and MP3 players) are used excessively, and disrupt the bedtime routine, this can lead to poorer sleep (see: Cain and Gradisar 2010).

In addition to the pointers here, various assessments are available (see: Appendix 5). These can help to identify simple changes to routine that might be a first stage in sorting out the problem.

Sleep hygiene has a number of specific aspects, and some examples are given in Table A3.

Table A3: Aspects of sleep hygiene

Aspects of sleep hygiene	Examples
Physiological	The person's drinking and eating pattern
Cognitive	Activities that affect level of mental activity and arousal before bed
Emotional	Activities that affect level of anger/arousal around bedtime
Sleep environment	Lights, music, television, the room temperature
Daytime sleep	Naps
Substance use	Alcohol, caffeine, recreational drugs
Physiological	Preparation for bed
Sleep stability	Variations in sleep pattern
Bed or bedroom sharing	Sharing with parent/s, sibling/s, other/s

Using Social Stories™ to encourage a good night-time routine

Social Stories are simple 'cartoon strip' picture sequences that can show the steps in everyday activities. They can be useful for explaining the sequence involved in going to bed (Gray and Garand 1993). Personalised Social Stories™ can be used to structure everyday activities, to provide a visual sequence reminder and help to establish a clear routine (see: Lorimer *et al.* 2002).

One study used a Social Story™, 'The Sleep Fairy', with four normal 2–7-year-old children (two boys and two girls). It reduced disruptive behaviour and established a better bedtime routine (Burke, Kuhn and Peterson 2004; Peterson and Peterson 2003).

Another study used a Social Story™ to help Peter, a 4-year-old boy. The Story™ was on laminated Velcro pages so it could be cleaned and any steps changed if needed (Table A4). Peter had ASD, severe learning disabilities, delayed language and behaviour problems. He had sleep difficulties and would only sleep in his parents' room with his mother close by. Peter took one to two hours to get to sleep and woke repeatedly through the night, waking early every morning. During the day his behaviour could be very difficult and both Peter and his mother were exhausted.

The plan was to get Peter to sleep in the lower bunk bed, in his own bedroom with his brother sleeping in the top bunk.

After introducing the Story™ at bedtime, Peter's night-time behaviour rapidly improved, continuing over a two-week period, except during a short illness. This was only one component of a broader behavioural intervention and it is impossible to say how much it contributed.

Table A4: Peter's Social Story™ outline

Sentence content	Pictures*
1. Peter's 'night, night' story	Thomas the Tank Engine Peter (close up)
2. My name is Peter... I cuddle down at night with Mum to read my 'night, night' story	Peter (close up) Mum with Peter on her lap reading story
3. This is me...this is my brother... this is our bedroom	Peter His brother Their bedroom
4. This me in my Bart pyjamas... I put my pyjamas on before 'night, night'	Peter in his pyjamas
5. This is my Thomas duvet, it's soft and cosy	Thomas the Tank Engine duvet
6. Tiger is my favourite toy, I bring him to bed with me	Tiger toy in Peter's bed
7. I bring my bottle to bed with me... When I have finished I put it down on the table	Peter with bottle in bed Bottle on table
8. Mum sits next to my bed to read me the 'night, night' story one last time	Mum sitting with a book next to Peter's bed
9. Here I am going to sleep on my own!	Peter in bed asleep
10. Good morning Peter... Mum wakes me with a hug and kiss for sleeping on my own	Mum opening curtains Mum (close up)
11. When I sleep on my own through the night, I get a Thomas sticker like this one to stick on my Thomas chart	Thomas the Tank Engine

*All pictures were cut out and Velcroed so Peter could order the pictures each time the book was read through.

Source: adapted from Moore 2004, Table 3, p.136. Copyright © 2004, John Wiley and Sons.

Having a clear bedtime routine can often help to improve children's sleep and make parents more confident. It can improve sleep, and maternal mood.

Sleep hygiene can be important but isn't always at the root of the problem. If it hasn't worked, you need to develop a treatment plan.

Deciding on your plan

Having kept a baseline diary, and put a good bedtime routine in place, if there is still a problem, the next stage is to focus on identifying the underlying problem, and decide what you need to do to sort it.

You should try to work on the various aspects that seem important from your evidence and continue with a diary record to monitor changes/improvements.

The following sections discuss different general approaches that are available for the major types of sleep problems and the evidence for them.

IN A NUTSHELL

Look at sleep hygiene, keep a baseline diary, make any obvious changes and see if this improves things. If the problem improves, great. However, if you still have a problem, you need to move on to see if you can pin it down and find a more specific solution.

— 7 —

WHY ARE SLEEP PROBLEMS MORE COMMON IN ASD?

How common are sleep problems in people with ASDs?

Sleep problems are more common in people with ASDs than in most other people. They are reported in over two-thirds of children and adolescents with ASD, compared to somewhere around 60% of developmentally delayed and 40% of normally developing controls. Nightmares and bedwetting seem to be particularly common, and are each seen in around one in three individuals. Behavioural insomnias (difficulties with settling to sleep) are the biggest single group, affecting around 60% of people with an ASD.

As the diagnostic criteria for both sleep problems and ASD change over time, and a number of assessment tools are used to assess sleep, it is not surprising that the precise results vary. Differences in the measures used can be important for whether problems are identified or go unnoticed, because different tools give different results. The results of actigraphy, for example, often disagree with other measures like videosomnography.

An overnight EEG can sometimes be a helpful assessment in getting to the root of the problem. EEGs can be difficult to carry out with children who have an ASD, as the procedure of applying the electrodes, although it shouldn't be painful or dangerous, can be uncomfortable and is often difficult to explain to the child. To help in carrying this out, structured preparation can considerably ease the process (see: Appendix 6).

Autistic children who sleep better (typically those who have more rapid eye movement (REM) or dream sleep) concentrate better when awake and get on better with others. With poorer sleep come higher levels of daytime problems, greater parental concerns and higher levels of stereotyped behaviours.

Parents of children with ASD often report that their children sleep for as long as others but with more sleeping difficulties and specific problems like fear of the dark, screaming and disoriented night-time waking (Tables A5 and A6).

Table A5: ASD sleep problems I

Sleep diagnosis	Number (N=59)	Percentage of total ASD group
None	9	15
Sleep-disordered breathing	1	2
Inadequate sleep hygiene	2	4
Parasomnias (linked to night-waking)	3	5
Insomnia of childhood – limit-setting type	6	10
Insomnia possibly due to medical condition (seizures (1); asthma (3); GERD (1))	6	10
Insomnia due to pervasive developmental disorder	11	19
No sleep problem – on active sleep medication*	11	19
Insomnia of childhood – sleep association type	12	20

GERD: Gastroesophageal reflux disease
* melatonin (4); catapres (clonidine) (1); risperidone (4); aripiprazole (2)
Source: data from Souders et al. 2009

Table A6: ASD sleep problems II

Sleep diagnosis	Number (N=477)	Percentage of total ASD group
Sleeps more than normal	67	14
Daytime sleepiness	100	21
Sleepwalking/Sleeptalking	167	35
Bedwetting	172	36
Nightmares	186	39
Sleeps less than normal	205	43
Waking too early	215	45
Frequent night-waking	238	50
Restless when asleep	267	56
Difficulty falling asleep	286	60

Source: data from Mayes et al. 2009

Do you really need to do anything about sleep problems?

Problems like nightmares and bedwetting can be distressing to the child and worrying and inconvenient to carers, and settling difficulties can be demanding and stressful. Are they likely to present more of a problem than this, or if untreated will they develop into anything worse?

Sleep problems in ASD appear to be linked to a number of other issues. They are associated with an increased severity of daytime behaviour problems, they are linked to greater social difficulties and they make learning more difficult. As they are more common in ASD and tend to be more severe and longer lasting, it is important that they are identified and treated.

In children with ASD, the presence of sleep problems more than doubles the liklihood of depression (Dominick *et al.* 2007). A number of studies have also shown a link between greater severity of autistic symptomology and poorer sleep (Schreck, Mulick and Rojahn 2003). Poor sleeping tends to be linked to increased sensory sensitivity, poorer social skills and increased levels of stereotyped movements (Schreck, Mulick and Smith 2004).

All of these suggest that sleep problems are linked to a range of other significant issues.

What sorts of things might make sleep problems more common in ASD?

Sleep problems are more common and more of an issue in ASD. We now know about several factors that can be involved:

1. Genetic differences can interfere with the production or metabolism of melatonin, an important chemical released by the pineal gland near the base of the brain that normally triggers sleep.

2. Disrupted development of cells called 'cortical interneurons' may be one early biological basis that could lead to problems with the sleep–wake cycle in ASD. These are small cells in the brain that are GABAergic (they are in pathways that use a neurotransmitter called gamma-aminobutyric acid).

Some ASDs may be 'developmental disconnection syndromes' (Geschwind and Levitt 2007). Here the normal connections between some brain regions have not fully formed, resulting in specific behavioural issues such as sleep disorders. This could explain, in some people at least, why sleep issues, seizure disorders and behavioural difficulties can go together.

3. People with autism are often less aware of others and of what they are doing (see, e.g.: Tager-Flusberg 1999). They can be less able to recognise and respond to bedtime cues and respond best to a clear night-time routine.

    The pattern of brain activity in autistic toddlers listening to 'bedtime stories' seems to be less and different from others (Redcay and Courchesne 2008).

    During bedtime stories one 3-year-old autistic toddler showed little activity in the left superior temporal gyrus. This is an important area for language processing. In contrast, other infants show bilateral increases with greater left hemisphere activity (Pierce 2011).

4. Poor sleep hygiene, and general behaviour management issues are common.

5. Sensory issues can make sleep problems worse.

6. Digestive problems can increase discomfort on lying down and make it harder to get to sleep, or cause you to wake because you are wet, soiled or needing the toilet. Reflux – when stomach acid comes up into the throat – worsens when someone lies down and is more common in people with ASD.

7. Side-effects of medication use: many medications can alter sleep patterns, and many psychostimulants, which are commonly used in ASD, suppress REM sleep. This interferes with growth hormone secretion, a process that occurs mainly during sleep. As a result, there can be a slowing of physical growth.

8. There could be an interaction between prescription medications.

9. There could be an interaction between prescription medications and diet, vitamin or mineral supplements.

Timing could provide a clue – did the problems start or worsen at the same time as any changes in things mentioned here – perhaps a new medication was being tried for seizures/ADHD/difficult behaviour? The person may have started consuming a new food or drink regularly (stimulant drinks can often affect the sleep pattern if taken to excess, and some children take over-the-counter stimulants to help them work for exams), you may have redecorated or installed stronger lights...

Even when more obvious biological factors are not part of the picture, the severity of sleep problems is associated with the severity of autistic symptoms – communication difficulties, stereotypes and overall severity are typically greater with more severe sleeping problems (see: Tudor, Hoffman and Sweeney 2012).

PART B

SPECIFIC SLEEP DIFFICULTIES

THE DIFFERENT SLEEP PROBLEMS, WHAT THEY ARE AND WHAT CAN HELP

Sleep disorders are often given limited emphasis in clinical training and the complexity of the issues is not well recognised. This was emphasised in a 2001 paper by the leading UK researcher on paediatric sleep problems, Gregory Stores, where he noted that the:

> diversity of sleep disorders is often not acknowledged in medical and other textbooks. Such inadequate coverage is part of the general neglect of the topic in professional training which persists despite the personal, social and economic importance of these disorders. (Stores 2001)

Internet searches provide easy access to information on many approaches that are proposed simply to help with 'sleep problems'. These are not usually ideal sources of information that might help you with the problem you are trying to fix. This is a bit like getting a garage to put petrol in your car because it has stopped working – if you have run out of fuel it is an excellent idea with a high probability of getting your car going again. If the car has stopped for a different reason (let's say the engine has seized or you have a flat battery) it doesn't matter how much fuel you put in or how often you repeat the process, it won't sort the problem. Trying an approach that works well for a different type of sleep problem may be using a well-evidenced and proven approach that is a complete waste of your time.

Where there is limited evidence on something with 'anecdotal support' it is a good idea to find out why there has been so little work rather than to dismiss out-of-hand something that seems sensible or plausible. The development of drugs for 'third world' diseases, before they were championed and supported by the Bill and Melinda Gates Foundation, was limited because there was little financial incentive to fund the research, not because it was known that medications were not effective or available. They weren't developed or marketed because they weren't thought to be commercially viable.

One example of an excellent treatment, if you happen to have the correct sleep problem, is melatonin supplementation. It has been intriguing to see the changing attitudes of many 'mainstream' clinicians to its use. Until fairly recently it was largely dismissed as a 'fad' supplement, available from herbalists and supplement shops, and viewed as used only by eccentric families.

Melatonin is now an over-the-counter medication (in the USA), and a licensed prescription medication (in the UK). Many doctors now prescribe it, and there is a steadily increasing literature on its use.

Melatonin can indeed help with sleep difficulties but only where the problem results from the body not making enough or an unusual pattern of melatonin release.

Unfortunately, people who develop problems don't tend to read the books first, and novel problems often present themselves. There is overlap across categories and a number of studies address more than one type of sleep difficulty.

The most common sleep difficulties in ASD

The most common sleep concerns reported are to do with sleeping for less time or less well than others. In Chapter 8, I have ordered these from the most to the least commonly reported difficulties.

As well as problems with sleep duration or quality, a number of other specific sleep problems are more common. These are covered in Chapter 9.

Various sleep and sleep-related problems are not overrepresented, but are just as common in ASD as in anyone else. These are covered in Chapter 10.

Some sorts of problems, although rare, can be difficult or distracting, while some are only more common in specific subgroups.

How sleep problems are classified

Sleep problems can be divided into two main groups: problems with sleeping (called 'dyssomnias') and problems around sleep (called 'parasomnias').

The common problems with sleeping are with getting to sleep, staying asleep or being sleepier during the day than normal. These are problems like delayed settling to sleep, frequent night-waking, early morning waking and excessive daytime sleepiness.

Most people with ASD who have sleep problems have difficulties in one or more of these areas.

The second group of sleep difficulties, the 'problems around sleep', are to do with things that occur during sleep. The main problems in this group are tooth-grinding, bedwetting, nightmares, night terrors, sleepwalking, sleeptalking and head-banging. A number of these are slightly more common in ASD than you would expect, but they are less common overall than sleeping problems.

When you have kept a baseline record, plot out your results and try to spot patterns. This can be particularly helpful if you find a regular but abnormal pattern or you see a changing picture with no obvious pattern. This will help you to decide what to do next. The most common patterns you might see are shown in Figure B1.

Putting your records into a graph can help you spot if this is a circadian rhythm sleep disorder. Delayed sleep phase disorder, advanced sleep phase disorder, non-24-hour sleep–wake syndrome and irregular sleep–wake rhythm are the most common of these (see: Barion and Zee 2007).

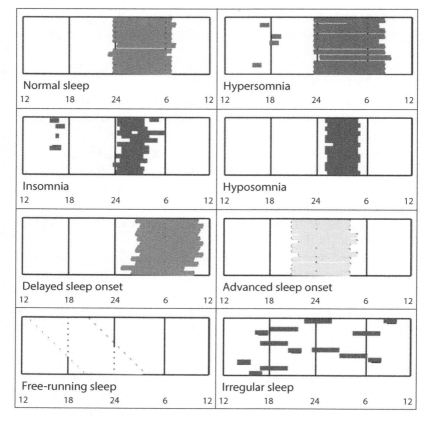

Figure B1: Typical records seen with different types of sleep difficulty
Source: based on Wulff, Porcheret, Cussans and Foster 2009

IN A NUTSHELL

There are a wide range of different sleep difficulties. Some can improve with time, some respond to simple changes to night-time routines, while others can need quite specialist interventions.

A clear idea of what sort of sleep problem someone has, whether it is likely to change over time and how bad it is, can help you to decide what to do next.

The rest of this section is divided into chapters and sections, each dealing with a specific sleep issue. Assuming that you have kept your sleep diary and identified a pattern, or that there is a specific issue like nightmares or bedwetting, you may be able to go directly to the appropriate section.

It is probably useful, even if you are now fairly sure of what you are dealing with, to check through the descriptions at the start of the other sections to make sure you are not missing anything.

— 8 —

DIFFICULTY GETTING TO SLEEP, STAYING ASLEEP, AND PROBLEMS WITH EXCESSIVE TIREDNESS

8.1 INSOMNIA

'Peter can't seem to get to sleep – we hear him up at all hours.'

Peter is a 12-year-old boy who has been diagnosed with Asperger syndrome. His parents say that he has always seemed to need less sleep than the rest of the family.

He sleeps in the same room as his brother Alan, who is 14. His brother is always asleep by 11pm on school nights while Peter is usually still awake well after 1am. Sometimes he is tired in the mornings, but he usually seems to get up without any difficulty at 7.15, the same time as his brother.

Peter has read that poor sleep can be linked to worse performance at school and has been repeatedly asking his parents to find out about help for him. He has no significant medical issues and is well placed at school. He has no active follow-up of his condition, having been discharged by the local hospital ASD team at the age of 7 once a school had been identified. No one from the team had mentioned that he might have sleep issues as part of his Asperger syndrome, and their family doctor had tended to play down the issue as common in boys and something he was likely to grow out of, whenever they had raised it with him. He suggested that from what he had read children with Aspergers were more likely to be anxious and Peter was probably worrying about nothing.

What is insomnia?

Insomnia is the term used for a persistent difficulty in getting to sleep or staying asleep. Typically by the time help is sought the symptoms will have been present for a month or more and they will be chronic. A general overview of insomnia can be found in Roth (2007).

Adults with insomnia are more likely to be anxious, depressed and suffer from persecutory ideation.

How common is it?

Insomnia is the most common sleep concern reported in ASD. A number of causes have been identified including neurochemical, psychiatric and behavioural factors (Miano and Ferri 2010; Silvia and Raffaele 2010). It is a frequent problem in Asperger syndrome (Tani *et al.* 2003, 2004).

It is also common throughout the population, with a lifetime prevalence of around 11%. One comparative study reported figures of over 15% in both Chinese and US children. In the USA, the prevalence of insomnia in adolescents aged 13–16 is around 9%.

The variations reported are probably because different assessments were used. Similar differences are even seen in longitudinal studies that use multiple assessment tools and data sources in tracking the same population.

Does it tend to get better anyway?

Once insomnia is chronic (after it has gone on for over a month) it is unlikely to improve without help. Rates of insomnia rise as people get older suggesting that age of onset varies but problems typically persist.

What can be done to treat it?

An early behavioural study focused on frequent night-waking in a group of seven infants aged 8–20 months. They used a four-week programme with two parts to it: 1) Parents were not to respond to their infant at night other than to check on them (but without talking to them) if they were worried, and 2) they were encouraged to establish a clear bedtime routine. Improvements were reported in all cases and maintained at both 3-month and 24-month follow-up checks (France and Hudson 1990).

A recent study of insomnia in three autistic children aged 8–9 (two boys and one girl) used weekly telephone contact and a handbook to help parents implement a three-component behavioural programme:

1. Faded bedtime (putting the child to bed slightly earlier each night).

2. Response–cost (rewards that could be gained or lost by achieving or failing to achieve bedtime targets).

3. Positive reinforcement (rewards for success).

All of the children went to sleep earlier and at three months this was maintained in two but more variable in the third child (Moon, Corkum and Smith 2010).

A number of studies have used cognitive-behavioural therapy (CBT) (see, e.g.: Espie and Kyle 2009). CBT is as effective as medication with a lower relapse rate (see: Riemann and Perlis 2009). Often its benefits can be complemented by medication and the combination can produce greater benefits than CBT alone. Although longer-term outcome data in children is lacking, this finding is well established in adults (Vallieres, Morin and Guay 2005).

A study on behavioural intervention in Angelman syndrome, focusing on a) better sleep hygiene, b) improved sleep-wake schedule, and c) reducing night-time parent–child interactions, reported significantly improved sleep patterns in five 2–11-year-old children with previously treatment-resistant sleep problems (Allen *et al.* 2013).

Melatonin

Melatonin is the only pharmacological treatment for insomnia with a robust children and adolescent evidence base. A review of melatonin treatment in 107 2–18-year-old children with ASD and insomnia (Andersen *et al.* 2008) reported 25% cured, 60% improved with ongoing sleep issues, 13% unchanged and one child's sleep as deteriorated, with outcome in one further child undetermined. Only three children were reported to have side-effects, all mild (including morning sleepiness and bedwetting). Most were also taking psychotropic medication.

Another small trial, in 7 out of an initial group of 11 ASD children, reported significantly increased time spent asleep and reduced night-time waking (Garstang and Wallis 2006).

In a study of 22 ASD children aged 3–16, whose sleep difficulties had not improved with behaviour management advice (Wright et al. 2011), melatonin improved both sleep latency (children falling asleep on average 47 minutes earlier) and time spent asleep (on average 52 minutes longer).

In Angelman Syndrome, low-dose melatonin elevates serum levels, reduces motor activity during sleep and improves sleep pattern (Zhdanova, Wurtman and Wagstaff 1999). In a randomised controlled trial (RCT) in eight children with this syndrome there was significant improvement, getting to sleep more quickly, spending longer asleep with reduced night-waking, with increased salivary melatonin levels (Braam et al. 2008).

The first large-scale RCT, in 146 children with ASD (Appleton et al. 2012; Gringras et al. 2012), looked at the effects of different dosages and the importance of baseline assessments. It recommended varied doses between 0.5 and 9mg as most effective and a minimum one-month baseline sleep diary before starting.

How likely is it to respond to treatment?

Various psychological treatments can help. Stimulus control, relaxation training, sleep restriction, cognitive-behavioural therapy (both with and without relaxation) and paradoxical intention have all been shown to work: 70–80% of those with insomnia can improve with these therapies. A subgroup achieve full remission, and medication can build on this.

Melatonin supplementation and melatonin receptor agonists are the only medications with promising results, and the data on these is preliminary. No robust evidence base shows clear benefit.

▬ Peter and his family were not reassured that this was probably nothing to worry about and had trawled the Internet for information on sleeping difficulties hoping to find a magic cure for his sleep problem. He had been put off the idea of having any sort of medicine to help him get to sleep and his view was reinforced by every story he seemed to come across reporting a bad reaction or an unexpected side-effect.

The family decided that they wanted to try a cognitive-behavioural approach. Peter was keen to go to a private therapist because the family knew a number of people working at the local NHS hospital department socially. Living in the UK, they were able to locate an appropriately qualified and registered therapist through the British Association for Behavioural and Cognitive Psychotherapy (BABCP: www.babcp.com).

Peter has been attending a therapist for regular weekly individual sessions over the past couple of months. He seems to be enjoying the sessions and has become much more organised about his evening routine – he has stopped doing homework reading in his bedroom, keeping his homework to the family study, and has a clearer night-time routine. He seems to be worrying less about his school performance and appears better rested and generally more confident. His family are not certain about the change in his sleep pattern but he seems to be worrying and talking less about it and they don't find him lying awake at night as often as before.

IN A NUTSHELL

There is good evidence for the effectiveness of behavioural and cognitive-behavioural approaches in the majority of people with insomnia. This is often improved on by the subsequent use of medication.

Preliminary evidence on melatonin suggests that it can be helpful, but currently it has a weaker evidence base than behavioural and cognitive-behavioural approaches.

Various other medications have some reported benefits but seem either only to have short-term benefits or to have a significant risk of causing side-effects.

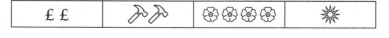

8.2 Difficulties with Settling to Sleep and Frequent Night-Waking

'He never goes down to bed and he's up and down like a yo-yo all night long.'

Jason is an able 5-year-old boy attending a mainstream school. He has difficulties making peer relationships, a number of obsessions and compulsions – he has memorised all of the football teams in the premier league and their match results for the last season. He recently received a diagnosis of ASD when his GP referred him for assessment. His family are concerned about his sleep pattern. Every evening they give him a shower and get him ready for bed at the same time as his younger sister Diana. When bedtime arrives, he always protests that he isn't tired and gets very upset when his parents try to take him to his room.

Most nights they relent and keep him up until he falls asleep on one of them and then they can carry him through to bed – often he wakes during this process and the settling period starts all over again.

During the night, Jason will typically waken his parents four or five times and unless one of them goes in to his bed to settle him he typically ends up sleeping with them from the early hours.

His parents argue a lot about how to deal with him. Often one of them (usually his dad) ends up sleeping on the couch.

What is 'difficulty getting to sleep'?

In infants this is a problem identified by parents or other carers. Many families have little to compare their baby against and, as there are large individual differences, few parents report worries. Many parents who raise worries are easily reassured, wanting to feel that the baby is 'normal'.

If you have an infant and are worried, try to check with someone with a range of experience, like a health visitor. Just because all of the other infants whose mums you are in contact with or who are in your extended family sleep more easily, this does not mean your infant has a problem.

Children often take longer falling asleep than we expect. Almost 60% of children have problems getting to sleep at least sometimes between the ages of 10 and 13 (Laberge *et al.* 2001).

What is 'frequent night-waking'?

There are differences in the reported extent and severity of night-waking depending on how it is assessed. Parental reports of night-waking differ from the results of actigraphy records (where a wristband worn by the infant monitors movement and wakenings). Different methods can give complementary pictures of sleep patterns that highlight aspects of the problem.

Night-waking tends to be more of an issue for parents in the early months (sometimes called the 'phase of sleep consolidation'). As young infants normally sleep with or beside their mothers it is not surprising that poor infant sleep patterns are more easily noticed.

Frequent night-waking is the most common sleep disorder seen in preschool children. As children get older, night-waking persists at the same frequency (there is wide variation, but the typical child will wake on average around twice each night) at least into early adolescence. As children get older they tend to self-console and return to sleep without alerting their parents, and parents are less likely to be around when this happens.

Do settling and waking problems tend to go together?

In younger children it is common for settling difficulties and night-waking problems, when they do happen, to occur together. Both problems are seen in around half of all children and can last through the preschool years.

These are fairly common problems and when they are present they tend to persist without specific help. When they are long-standing, this can affect development, and it should be a key target for early intervention (Sadeh and Sivan 2009).

How common are they?

Problems getting to sleep are perhaps the most commonly reported sleeping problem at all ages. By around 3 months parents report that around 30% of infants are not sleeping through the night. Persistent night-waking is common in small children and is thought to affect around a quarter of all children between 1 and 5.

In ASD these are also the most prevalent issues reported by parents of those with ASD, in 50–60% of cases (Mayes *et al.* 2009).

In one study of 4–10-year-olds (Souders *et al.* 2009), around a quarter of the ASD children but only 1 in 20 controls had frequent night-waking. Settling to sleep also took longer in the ASD group. 'Behavioural insomnia sleep-onset type' was the most common type of difficulty, in around 1 in 5 ASDs.

Do they tend to get better anyway?

It is surprising, given how commonly these problems are reported, that the evidence on treatment is quite limited.

These problems are common through the preschool years, being seen in around 40% of all babies and toddlers. They tend to continue once established, and the age they begin at is variable.

What can be done to treat them?

Various parent-implemented programmes can be effective. Success depends on finding an approach that you can follow consistently, that targets the specific problem and that is acceptable to all concerned.

These are common problems, they can be distressing to deal with, but are not harmful and will usually respond quite quickly to a consistent approach. Try not to worry, decide what you feel comfortable doing, and be consistent – give the child the message that you are calm, consistent, reassuring and in control, not panicking, unpredictable and difficult to understand.

Research with preschoolers shows that both behavioural interventions and medication have beneficial effects in the short term. Longer-term benefits have only been shown for behavioural interventions.

Start by keeping a sleep diary. In one study, 85% of parents reported that the problems settled after getting some basic information about sleep in childhood and keeping a diary, even before they had tried any type of intervention.

Having a clear bedtime routine and dealing with issues quickly and quietly can often reduce settling issues, night-time crying and tantrums.

One small study used a bedtime 'pass' that the child could exchange to leave their bedroom briefly after bedtime (Friman *et al.* 1999). The pass reduced both crying and how often they left their room and gave the child a feeling of control and a more acceptable way to achieve it.

Children can also learn their night-time routine by using a bedtime Social Story™. Social Stories™, described in Part A, can be effective for a range of issues. They are effective with sleep problems in most 2–7-year-olds (Burke, Kuhn and Peterson 2004). They also work with ASD (Peterson and Peterson 2003; Burke, Kuhn and Peterson 2004).

Another behavioural approach is called 'faded bedtime with response cost'. This was tried with four children, all with learning problems, self-injury, ASD and night-time sleeping problems. Two also had excessive daytime sleepiness (Piazza and Fisher 1991).

There are two parts to the approach:

1. Gradually make bedtime earlier (the 'faded bedtime' part).

2. Take the child out of bed and keep them awake for an hour if they haven't fallen asleep quickly when put to bed. This is repeated until the child falls asleep.

All four children improved and the improvement was maintained. The authors extended their work, comparing it to a 'bedtime schedule' in two groups of similar childen. They reported that the faded bedtime approach had better results (Piazza, Fisher and Scherer 1997). A further paper has described its successful use with a 2-year-old girl, treated by her parents (Ashbaugh and Peck 1998).

Mothers given advice on handling 6–12-month-old infant sleep difficulties reported initial improvements (Hiscock and Wake 2002). The sleep problems and the amount of improvement correlated with the mother's level of depressed mood – when the sleep difficulties eased, the mothers reported being less depressed. Although improved mood was maintained, improved sleep was not. Even earlier intervention may be needed to produce sustained benefit.

'Planned ignoring' was used for disruptive night-time behaviour in four children with developmental disorders including a 6.5-year-old boy with ASD (Didden et al. 2002). All improved and this was maintained for a five-month follow-up.

Fear of the dark is a different issue, and can be dealt with in the same way as other sorts of fears and phobias – gradually getting them used to the situation with images and inducing feelings related to being in darkness. This is called 'systematic desensitisation'. It might involve working through a series of stages – the child goes from sleeping earlier with a light on in the room, gradually going to bed later with the room being made progressively darker – installing a dimmer switch can help with this. This gradual change can be paired with rewards for success and encouraging them to use positive self-statements, like 'I am brave and I can take care of myself when I'm alone or in the dark', if they start to feel anxious.

Jodi Mindell (1999) reviewed 41 studies on behavioural treatment for bedtime refusal and night-time waking. The studies she reviewed reported good overall success but much of the literature was noted to be poorly documented.

There has been only one randomised controlled study of medication for night-waking problems in 1–3-year-olds using trimeprazine (alimemazine). Those treated were reported as waking up less and spending less time awake at night, with longer periods of night-time sleep than controls (Simonoff and Stores 1987).

How likely are they to respond to treatment?

There is good evidence for a number of approaches:

- extinction
- graduated extinction
- positive routines and faded bedtime
- scheduled awakening
- parent education and prevention
- interventions to reduce night-time fears.

These improve family functioning in addition to their effects on sleep. The strongest evidence is for two main approaches:

1. Planned ignoring (both extinction and graduated extinction) can be effective and is usually easy to implement.

2. Positive bedtime routines (improved sleep hygiene).

These treatments work in around 70% of cases.

Better research is needed and so far there have been no good randomised controlled trials of different treatments for settling and night-waking problems.

These issues appear to be around five times more common in ASD, but there is no evidence on the relative effectiveness of specific approaches with ASD.

Table B1 is a representative selection of studies on treatment of settling and night-waking problems.

Table B1: Settling and night-waking studies

Approach	Reported population	Outcome	Follow-up	Issues	Source references
Withdrawal of reinforcement for problem behaviour	19 under 5-year-olds	17/19 improved, 16/19 maintained at follow-up	6 months		Jones and Verduyn (1983)
Alimemazine tartrate	18/50 1–3-year-olds	Reduced waking, longer sleep	Not reported	Cardiac instability Respiratory depression	Simonoff and Stores (1987)
Systematic ignoring (SyI)	Infants and toddlers, 6–54 months 11 SyI 11 scheduled waking (SW) 11 non-intervention control	SyI=SW> Control	3 and 6 weeks		Rickert and Johnson (1988)
Faded bedtime with response cost protocol	4 children, LD, self-injury + ASD	Improvements in all	Variable from 1 month to 1 year		Piazza and Fisher (1991)
Faded bedtime with response cost protocol	Developmentally normal 2-year-old toddler	Improvement	1 month		Ashbaugh and Peck (1998)
Standard ignoring (StI) and graduated ignoring (GI)	16–48-month-olds 16 StI; 17 GI; 16 list control	StI=GI> Control	2 months		Reid, Walter and O'Leary (1999)
Written information and 'controlled crying'	76 6–12-month-olds and 76 controls	53 vs 36/76 improved at 2 months but not sustained	2 and 4 months		Hiscock and Wake (2002)
Social Stories™	4 normal 2–7-year-olds	Night-waking resolved in all, better night-time behaviour	3 months		Burke, Kuhn and Peterson (2004)

■— Jason's parents wanted to try 'planned ignoring' as the easiest strategy to implement. They explained to him that there were new rules about bedtime and that he had to be in his room before he fell asleep and to stay in his room quietly until the morning unless he needed to get up to go to the toilet. If he was noisy and woke his sister, he would not get more storytime and would miss his reward in the morning – they had bought a sticker chart for his local football team and this was stuck up above his bed. This idea was linked with the promise of a reward if he managed to succeed.

The first night, Jason went to his room with sister Diana and they listened to their mother read them a bedtime story. By the end of the story, Diana was fast asleep and was settled down in bed by Mum but Jason was still wide awake. Mum reminded him that he was to try to stay quietly in his room, but he was still wide awake when she left. He lasted 20 minutes before creeping downstairs saying he was bored and couldn't get to sleep. His mum repeated the process, reading to him, reminding him about staying in his bed and leaving the room saying she would check on him in half an hour and read to him some more if he hadn't come out. To her amazement when she checked on him half an hour later, he had dozed off on his bed and she was able to get him under his covers without waking.

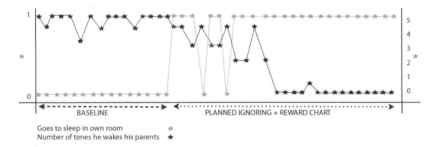

Goes to sleep in own room ☆
Number of times he wakes his parents ★

Figure B2: Jason's sleep pattern

From their baseline diaries, they had hoped that he might manage 20 minutes before coming through (usually he could be quiet in the living room for periods of 20 minutes or so after his sister went to bed, and this had been set as the target for getting his first sticker. His first night excelled their expectations and was a strong incentive for Jason and his parents to continue once they saw he was capable of improvement.

So Jason was systematically ignored for being noisy and out of his room after bedtime (*planned ignoring*), he had a clear routine around going to bed (*improved sleep hygiene*), and this was coupled with a reward system for progressive improvement (*positive reinforcement*), which increased his motivation to comply with what he was being asked to do.

IN A NUTSHELL

Difficulties settling and frequent night-waking are common problems in young children. They are five times more common in ASD.

There is a good chance that these problems will persist unless treated, but most will respond to the fairly simple strategies of improving sleep hygiene and planned ignoring.

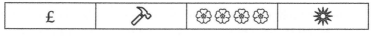

8.3 Restless Sleepers

There are several different reasons someone can seem restless while asleep. These are thought to have different causes and might require different solutions.

'Restless legs syndrome' and 'periodic limb movements in sleep' are covered in the first section. 'Sleep-related rhythmic movement disorder' is covered in the third. It is currently viewed as a separate disorder, however it is similar in presentation to the others and its management is similar. For all there is a reasonably high spontaneous improvement rate. Improvements are reported with several medications. Some cases are linked to problems with iron metabolism and can benefit from supplementation.

Sleep can also be restless in someone having 'nocturnal seizures', covered in 8.3.ii. These can present in a number of different ways, from bedwetting, sleepwalking and making continuous high-pitched noises (called 'stridor'), to choking. Some night-time seizures are harmless but many require specific medical treatment.

REM sleep behaviour disorder is a condition in which the person affected is physically active during rapid eye movement sleep.

8.3.I RESTLESS LEGS SYNDROME

▬ **'Fidgity Philip – he never seems to stop.'**

Philip is a 10-year-old boy with 'high-functioning autism'. He has a long-standing problem – he has always been described by his family as a very restless sleeper. He is often found with his duvet in a pile on the floor in the morning. His parents have on several occasions gone into his room and found him fast asleep with his legs jerking repeatedly in an odd way and have been worrying these may have been epileptic fits. His doctor referred him to the local paediatric neurologist for review who arranged an admission for an overnight EEG. While the EEG was being recorded he had a prolonged leg-jerking episode – the EEG showed no evidence of seizure activity.

What is restless legs syndrome?

RLS (restless legs syndrome) was first described by the English physician Thomas Willis in 1672. The Swedish neurologist Karl-Axel Ekbom published a clear account of the condition in 1945. It is sometimes called Willis-Ekbom disease.

RLS and periodic limb movement disorder in sleep (PLMDS)/ sleep-related rhythmic movement disorder (SRMD) are currently seen as separate conditions. Both involve abnormal leg movements during sleep. In RLS, the movements are said to be the cause of disagreeable sensations, while those in PLMDS/SRMD are not. RLS is seen in parents of those diagnosed with both RLS and PLMDS/SRMD, and they seem likely to have a common genetic basis (Picchietti *et al.* 2009).

The Pediatric Restless Legs Syndrome Severity Scale (P-RLS-SS) © can be used to get a clear picture of RLS in 6–18-year-olds (Arbuckle *et al.* 2010). This was intended for use as a research tool but may be useful to monitor improvement.

Both RLS and PLMDS are described as different from SRMD (see under 8.2.iii below), however the latter two seem almost identical. It is not clear whether any of the differences between these groups are important, or if they are part of the same condition.

How common is it?

Based on two large studies, the conditions are extremely common. RLS has been reported to affect 1-in-20 to 1-in-50 people and PLMDS around 1-in-25.

Does it tend to get better anyway?

RLS is a lifelong disorder that can worsen with age but may go through periods of remission. Forty per cent of affected adults report similar symptomology to those in childhood (Picchietti and Stevens 2008).

There is currently no information on the natural history of untreated PLMDS.

What can be done to treat it?

RLS tends to get worse when sleep is poor. Try to ensure a good sleep routine and that sleep hygiene is as good as possible.

A range of basic strategies are recommended:

- Avoid substances and medications that tend to make symptoms worse (the usual culprits are nicotine, caffeine and alcohol).

- Limit access to mentally alerting activities in the hour or so before bedtime (things like computer games; crosswords, etc.).

- Use cognitive-behavioural strategies similar to those used in insomnia (Pigeon and Yurcheshen 2009; Silber et al. 2004).

Elemental iron

Iron regulates the activity of dopamine in the body and there is evidence for low iron levels in RLS (Kryger, Otake and Foerster 2002; Simakajornboon et al. 2003). Where iron levels are low, long-term benefits have been reported with supplementation of 3mg of *elemental* iron per day (Simakajornboon et al. 2006).

The percentage of elemental iron varies markedly by the type of iron supplement used – ferrous gluconate contains only 12% elemental iron while ferrous fumarate is roughly 33% and a carbonyl iron supplement is 100% elemental. This means that a 3mg carbonyl iron supplement would provide enough elemental iron, while 25mg of ferrous gluconate would be needed. This is important because excessive iron ingestion can cause problems, and in large amounts can be toxic. As a number of foods such as breads, flours and cereals are now fortified with iron, it is important to check a) that the person is low in elemental iron and b) the total amount ingested will not exceed safe levels (see: Murphy 1974).

A report on a 12-week RCT with 28 patients found that, in contrast to the reports on its beneficial effects in PLMDS, ferrous sulphate was ineffective in the management of RLS symptoms (Davis et al. 2000).

Dopamine agonists

Ropinirole is a generic dopamine agonist. It is approved in the USA for the treatment of RLS. A recent systematic review (Erichsen, Ferri and Gozal 2010) concluded it is safe and effective in the management of both RLS and PLMDS.

Other dopamine agonists such as rotigotine show significant benefits in RLS (see, e.g.: Hogl *et al.* 2010). Rotigotine has not been approved for use by people younger than 18, but is currently showing good results in older age groups (see: Merlino *et al.* 2009).

The lack of a biological marker for RLS, and until recently the lack of criteria for assessing effects of dopamine augmentation, have hampered developments in this area (see: Garcia-Borreguero and Williams 2010).

In a series of seven paediatric cases with RLS/PLMDS and comorbid ADHD, dopamine agonists such as pergolide and the naturally occurring dopamine precursor l-DOPA were shown to benefit children who had responded poorly to stimulant medication (Walters *et al.* 2000).

A number of medications now have evidence to support their use in RLS, the main treatments to date being levodopa, ropinirole, pramipexole, cabergoline, pergolide and gabapentin.

How likely is it to respond to treatment?

There are few studies to date and differences reported may not be treatment specific. A large number of treatments have been tried. Some have good reported results and good long-term outcomes as with Simakajornboon *et al.*'s 2006 paper on two-year follow-up on elemental iron in RLS.

In general, untreated RLS is lifelong. There can be periods of remission but it tends to worsen over time. Current therapies can control symptoms in most cases.

■— Oliver's family have been very worried about his persistent night-time problems. Having spent days trawling the Internet and asking other families for advice on 'chatrooms', they felt as bemused as ever – they had even more options and no clear guidance.

Oliver has had a review at the neurology clinic, where they looked through the EEG recorded during the episode that happened while he was in hospital. This reassured them that Oliver did not have a seizure disorder. They were told that Oliver had a working diagnosis of 'restless legs syndrome'.

The family completed a sleep hygiene assessment and a number of aspects of his bedtime routine have been improved. He is getting to sleep at a more regular time and starting to sleep for longer. They were surprised at the number of stimulants in his normal diet – he was keen on a number of drinks that are high in caffeine, and have limited these to times before 6pm.

A dietician looked through a diet diary kept on Oliver's food and drink intake over a couple of weeks. In addition to the high levels of stimulants and refined sugar he had been taking, she pointed out that he also had a diet that had low levels of a number of essential minerals, including iron. She gave them advice on foods with higher mineral content and suggested an iron supplement.

He had been playing games on his computer before going to bed that seemed to make him quite agitated – he is now allowed time on these between returning home and the evening meal but not later at night.

The family are not keen to consider medication and have noticed improvements in his level of agitation and in his sleeping since changing his diet and night-time routine.

IN A NUTSHELL

There is a limited amount of evidence on what works for RLS.

- Try to avoid or limit caffeine, nicotine and alcohol intake.

- Check iron levels and correct these if they are low.

- Try to have a quiet hour leading up to bedtime.

- Consider CBT if this is available and the person has the verbal ability to make use of it.

- There is some limited evidence for benefits from various medications that alter central nervous system (CNS) dopamine levels – medication is not currently part of a treatment package of choice but it may be worth rechecking the evidence on this.

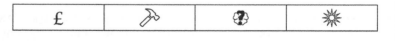

8.3.II NOCTURNAL SEIZURES

— 'He gets hot and sweaty, shakes in his sleep, and usually wets his bed. We can always tell when one is coming.'

Hector is a 7-year-old boy with autism and mild learning difficulties. He has always been a restless sleeper, so much so that his parents tend to take him into bed with them so he does not disturb his brothers. He has a history of febrile convulsions, having had a number of fits when he was smaller that were brought on by high temperatures. Typically these happened when he had an ear infection and was running a high temperature. The family were reassured that he was unlikely to develop epilepsy and no medication was prescribed, but they were told that there was an increased possibility that he might develop fits.

Recently there have been a number of episodes when his parents have gone in to check on him last thing at night and found him jerking oddly in his sleep. The episodes have been quite brief, lasting at most 30 seconds or so, and on a couple of these times they have found that he has wet his bed. Hector is very upset at the bedwetting but does not seem to have any awareness of having had the convulsions. On one occasion he had bitten through the side of his tongue and bled quite profusely.

What are nocturnal seizures?

Nocturnal seizures are epileptic fits occurring during sleep. A useful review can be found in Bazil (2004).

They can worsen if there is another sleep disorder like obstructive sleep apnoea (OSA) and can improve when it is controlled (Hollinger et al. 2006). In a recent study, 14.2% of 127 child OSA cases had paroxysmal EEG activity consistent with seizures (Miano et al. 2009).

Night-time seizures can be recognised in various ways:

- stridor (a wheezing sound made when breathing)

- episodic nocturnal wandering (a form of sleepwalking)

- choking.

Some nocturnal seizures are harmless and improve without treatment (Panayiotopoulos et al. 2008), others do not. Management should be on a case-by-case basis, looking out for possible treatment side-effects (Oguni 2011). When nocturnal seizures are suspected, it is important that these are diagnosed/excluded by a clinician with relevant experience.

EEGs commonly show epileptiform abnormalities in ASD. When 889 patients were routinely given EEGs over a nine-year period (Chez *et al.* 2006), more than 60% showed evidence of epileptiform activity. There were no previous diagnoses within this group of epilepsy, any genetic condition, or a CNS malformation. Abnormal EEGs were also seen in the non-autistic non-epileptic siblings of 12 and in a small number of the 162 typically developing non-sibling controls (Chez *et al.* 2004). Abnormal activity was most often noted over the right temporal lobe. An abnormal sleep EEG was not associated with behavioural regression.

Giannotti *et al.* (2008) compared EEGs from 34 regressive and 70 non-regressive ASD cases and found greater EEG abnormalities linked to regression.

A number of genetic conditions that can cause seizure activity are more common in ASD (see: Aitken 2010a).

Occasionally people have 'non-epileptic' seizures with similar behaviour but no EEG abnormality. These can occasionally happen in sleep and were reported in 1% of a sample of over 2000 investigated for nocturnal seizures (Orbach, Ritaccio and Devinsky 2003).

Epileptic and non-epileptic movement disorders in sleep can be discriminated (Tinuper *et al.* 2007). EEG videotelemetry is the best method of doing this, but where this is not feasible, factors like the presence of stridor, choking and sleepwalking, the age at onset, and number, timing and duration of episodes can often help.

How common are they?

No one knows exactly how common nocturnal seizures are, but they are rare. The extent of the overlap with ASD is not clear and has rarely been investigated (Manni and Terzaghi 2010).

In many cases successful treatment of seizures improves sleep problems (Tachibana *et al.* 1996). Conversely, some medications used to treat epilepsy may cause or exacerbate sleep difficulties (see: Bazil 2003).

Circadian rhythm differences can affect seizure control, but the nature and strength of this effect is poorly understood (Hofstra and de Weerd 2009).

Do they tend to get better anyway?

Benign seizures typically improve over time and do not leave lasting problems.

The risk of progression from nocturnal to daytime seizures seems to be between 0% and 19%. There is a better than 4 in 5 chance that someone with nocturnal seizures will not develop daytime seizures.

What can be done to treat them?

The treatments of choice, and whether they will help, depend on the type of nocturnal seizures. As with any form of epilepsy, treatment should be with the advice and supervision of a competent and appropriately accredited doctor.

Several types of epilepsy cause nocturnal seizures. Three are most common and account for most cases:

1. benign Rolandic epilepsy

2. nocturnal frontal lobe epilepsy (NFLE)

3. generalised tonic-clonic seizures.

A fourth type, 'nocturnal tonic seizures', are typically seen in Lennox-Gastaut syndrome. Nocturnal tonic seizures happen during non-rapid eye movement (NREM) sleep and can be harder to control (see discussion in Camfield and Camfield 2002).

Seizures and sleep disorders can both can be associated with low melatonin and, as with some sleep issues, improvements in seizure disorders have been reported with melatonin supplements (Bazil *et al.* 2000; Fauteck *et al.* 1999).

Certain sorts of sleep problem are more common in epilepsy. OSA is seen in 20% of children with epilepsy (Kaleyias *et al.* 2008), and seizure control can improve with OSA treatment. The association may be due to restrictions on exercise, or an effect of seizure medication. Gabapentin, pregabalin, sodium valproate, vigabatrin and carbamazepine have all been implicated in weight gain (see: Ben-Menachem 2007).

How likely are they to respond to treatment?

Outcome is largely dependent on seizure type.

In benign Rolandic epilepsy, most improve during puberty without treatment – the person outgrows the disorder. In most cases, a good outcome is predictable without treatment and no anti-epileptic medication is required (Peters, Camfield and Camfield 2001).

In NFLE, around 70% of cases are well controlled on medication with good seizure control, improved sleep and a good developmental outcome. Where medication is ineffective, improvement has been shown after surgical removal of the focus (Nobili *et al.* 2007). No long-term surgical case follow-up is yet available.

Generalised tonic-clonic seizures are harder to control and have a poorer outcome (Rantala and Putkonen 1999). In some cases improvements have been reported on a ketogenic diet (see, e.g.: Calandre, Martinez-Martin and Campos-Castellano 1978). It's called ketogenic because compounds called ketones are excreted in the urine on a low carbohydrate diet.

▬ Hector's parents have recently gone back to the paediatrician in their local hospital with concerns about his nocturnal seizures. She has agreed to refer him to the neurology service for further assessment and he is to have an overnight admission for sleep recording.

As Hector is pre-pubertal, they want to be sure about the diagnosis before considering the right course of treatment, as the outcomes are so variable; some are benign and others have serious consequences if they are not treated.

IN A NUTSHELL

Assessment and treatment of seizure-related sleep issues requires professional assistance to identify the type of epilepsy, the need for treatment and the most appropriate approach when treatment is required. A number of approaches can be successful in more complex cases, but should not be embarked on without appropriate support and guidance.

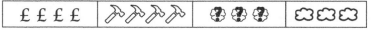

| £ £ £ £ | 🔨🔨🔨🔨 | 🌀🌀🌀 | ⌷⌷⌷ |

8.3.III SLEEP-RELATED RHYTHMIC MOVEMENT DISORDER/PERIODIC LIMB MOVEMENT DISORDER

▬ 'Why on earth does he keep doing that?'

James is an 8-year-old boy with a diagnosis of Asperger syndrome. He is a bright boy but has always had difficulty concentrating in school and is being assessed for ADHD because his teachers feel that he is 'underachieving' academically.

Pete, his 6-year-old brother, has recently started sharing a room with James as their 2-year-old baby sister now needs her own bedroom. The family always knew that James was a restless sleeper but, recently, since they have been going in and checking on his younger brother, his parents have become concerned because they have observed unusual jerking movements of his legs on several occasions while he is sound asleep. His mother was a general nurse and has seen epileptic fits in adult patients and they are worried that James may be having seizures during his sleep.

He has become more tired recently and complains about having 'sore muscles' in his legs.

Current classifications discriminate between sleep-related rhythmic movement disorder (SRMD), restless legs syndrome (RLS) and periodic limb movement disorder in sleep (PLMDS). There is a significant degree of overlap between all of these classifications. The genetic research shows a heightened risk of SRMD or RLS in children with a parent diagnosed as having RLS (see: Picchietti *et al.* 2009). The literature tends to treat SRMD as a separate condition, but given their obvious similarities, we will combine the information on SRMD and PLMDS.

What is sleep-related rhythmic movement disorder?

In SRMD there are stereotyped repetitive rhythmic movements. These typically involve the head and neck and happen either while going to sleep or once sleeping. They typically take the form of head-banging (sometimes called jacatio capitis nocturna), head-rolling or body-rocking.

The term periodic limb movement disorder of sleep (PLMDS) has been used in describing the same clinical features (Crabtree *et al.* 2003).

An association between SRMD/PLMDS and attention-deficit hyperactivity disorder (ADHD) is reported in a high proportion of cases, with around 45% being comorbid (Stepanova, Nevsimalova and Hanusova 2005).

In some, the pattern may be complex and involve different stereotyped movements. These can appear to be seizures but have a normal EEG (Su *et al.* 2009). They are classified as sleep-related movement disorder on the ICSD-2.

How common is it?

In infancy, stereotyped movements during sleep are common, and seen in up to 59%, dropping to around 5% by age 5 (discussed in Mayer, Wilde-Frenz and Kurella 2007). Persistent SRMD/PLMDS at older ages is typically only seen in either people with ASD or learning disabilities (see: Newell *et al.* 1999).

Does it tend to get better anyway?

The majority improve in early childhood, typically before school. In older cases the problem is likely to require treatment. A study that classified a series of clinical SMRD/PLMDS cases found 20 out of 24 were male, with a family history in only two (Mayer *et al.* 2007).

Persistent SMRD/PLMDS may be more common with comorbid ADHD (Stepanova *et al.* 2005).

The possibility of comorbidity with ADHD has been little studied because on the DSM system, until the most recent revision, autism and ADHD could not be diagnosed in the same person so the association could not be reported.

What can be done to treat it?

A recent study (Picchietti and Picchietti 2008) recommends reviewing sleep hygiene, using the 'Peds RLS NEWREST' chart as a reminder:

BOX B1: THE PEDS RLS NEWREST CHART: TIPS FOR BETTER SLEEP

N **N**utritional needs. A healthy age-appropriate diet should be adopted. Any foods containing caffeine, such as chocolate, and drinks such as soda, energy drinks, iced tea and coffee should be restricted, especially in the late afternoon and evening. Current dietary iron intake and the need for iron supplementation should be assessed.

E **E**nvironment for sleeping. The bedroom should be relaxing, quiet and only for sleeping. Find another room for studying, loud music, TV and 'timeout'.

W **W**atch for and report restlessness, uncomfortable leg sensations and disturbed sleep, especially when these affect daytime function.

R **R**egular sleep schedule with a routine bedtime and wake-up time even on weekends.

E **E**xercise daily. Physical activity can reduce RLS sensations and increases deep sleep.

S **S**top substance use that interferes with good sleep such as tobacco, alcohol and recreational drugs.

T **T**ake prescribed medicine and/or approved iron supplements consistently.

Source: adapted from Picchietti and Picchietti 2008, Table 5, p.59. Copyright © 2008, Elsevier.

When associated with sleep apnoea, if the apnoea improves, improvements are often seen in the movements (Chirakalwasan *et al.* 2009).

SRMD/PLMDS can worsen with low serum ferritin and on treatment with antidepressants or antihistamines. Iron levels should be checked and, where low, corrective supplements should be given (Simakajornboon *et al.* 2003). Consistent long-term benefits on PLMDS are reported using 3mg of elemental iron per day in children with low blood levels (<50ng per ml) (Simakajornboon *et al.* 2006). Low serum ferritin is reported in a high proportion of autistic cases (Dosman *et al.* 2006), and supplementation seems generally helpful in managing sleep disorders (Dosman *et al.* 2007).

Benefits of iron supplementation may result from its role as an essential co-factor for the enzyme tyrosine hydroxylase in dopamine production. Dopamine is one of the main neurotransmitters (Earley *et al.* 2000).

One review of treatments used up to 2003 found only a few single case reports of the use of conventional medications, with some claims of symptomatic control with low-dose clonazepam (Hoban 2003).

Dopamine agonists (drugs that increase levels of dopamine or of dopaminergic activity) such as ropinirole have also been reported to be helpful (see: Erichsen *et al.* 2010), however there is very limited information on the use, benefit or side-effects of dopamine agonists with this group.

How likely is it to respond to treatment?

A helpful recent overview of outcomes can be found in Bonnet *et al.* (2010).

The majority of cases improve during childhood. Even without improvement, the person's intelligence and overall development seem unaffected (Mayer *et al.* 2007).

In rare cases where symptoms persist into adulthood, they typically head bang and/or body roll (Stepanova *et al.* 2005).

Where investigated with video telemetry, persistent cases often show unusual EEG patterns at 0.5–2.0 Hz (Manni and Terzaghi 2010). This suggests either comorbidity with epilepsy or that the movements themselves indicate seizure activity. No studies have as yet reported on treating SRMD/PLMDS with anti-epileptic medication.

James has been admitted for an overnight videotelemetry study and his family have been reassured by discussing with their neurologist and from reading the available papers that he is unlikely to have any lasting problems as a result of his sleep movements.

He has been started on a course of mineral supplements to try to help with his sore leg muscles, but otherwise he and his parents feel confident that he is more than likely to grow out of the movements and, as they do not disturb his younger brother and James is not troubled by them, the family are happy to live with them at present.

IN A NUTSHELL

Explore ferritin levels and possible treatments to help with muscular discomfort.

When epilepsy has been excluded as a possible alternative cause, the presentation is not worrying, and most cases will improve without specific treatment.

SRMD is benign and does not seem to affect development even when the problems have persisted into adulthood.

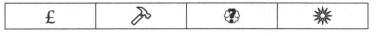

8.3.IV REM SLEEP BEHAVIOUR DISORDER (RSBD)

▬ 'The boy who fought with his dreams.'

Tom was only referred for help at the age of 13 but had always been a restless sleeper. He is a bright, articulate boy with an Asperger diagnosis who has difficulties with peer relationships and accepting boundaries but is progressing well academically. Ever since he was a toddler, his parents have been used to finding his duvet in a heap across the room and Tom sweating and shivering, fast asleep, at the edge of his bed. His grandparents said that Tom's father was like that and had just grown out of it so it was probably nothing to worry about.

Recently, the family have found that most evenings they hear Tom thrashing about in the middle of the night more often and more loudly as if he is fighting with something or somebody. When they question him about these times, he tells them about his dreams. These often have the same theme, in which Tom is being chased through a dark forest by wild animals and he has to hit out at them to keep them at bay. During these 'dream fights' Tom has broken a number of things, usually by throwing objects at his imaginary pursuers, smashing things like his DVD player and alarm clock against the wall.

What is REM sleep behaviour disorder?

In RSBD, the normal loss of muscle control seen in REM sleep doesn't happen. Rather than merely dreaming/imagining what is happening, the person exhibits complex motor behaviour while dreaming, apparently acting out their dreams (see: Paparrigopoulos 2005; Boeve 2010).

RSBD is typically a condition seen in older men, but it is also seen in children with autism.

Thirumalai, Shubin and Robinson (2002) described RSBD in 5 of 12 ASD children assessed because of sleep disruption and nocturnal awakening.

RSBD is often missed in clinical practice unless specific questions are asked about the nature of the behavioural events during sleep (Frauscher *et al.* 2010).

Diagnosis requires:

1. an EEG pattern usually seen during REM sleep, but without the normal loss of muscular control (called atonia)

and one of the following:

2a. a history of sleep-related injurious, potentially injurious or disruptive behaviours (where descriptions are given by parents or partners of behaviour consistent with acting out their dreams)

or:

2b. observation of such behaviour during polysomnography recording

and:

3. no epileptic activity recorded during REM sleep (unless periods of RSBD can be clearly distinguished from any concurrent REM sleep-related seizure disorder and both types of pattern are present).

In addition:

4. no alternative explanation (such as another sleep disorder; a separate medical, neurological or mental disorder; a medication effect; some form of substance abuse).

An older man, in 'The Man Who Fought in Sleep' (Budhiraja 2007), could clearly describe having dreams in which he was fighting with animals or monsters. Some of the episodes occurred during polysomnography-corroborated REM sleep, at which time he was seen to be kicking, punching and shouting at his partner.

Half of those diagnosed with narcolepsy (discussed later in section 10.5) show the same pattern of REM sleep muscle activity as is seen in RSBD (Dauvilliers *et al.* 2007).

How common is it?

This is not clearly established. The report of Thirumalai *et al.* (2002) suggests that in ASD children with disturbed sleep RSBD may be more common than previously realised.

As most children and adolescents sleep alone, RSBD may go unnoticed unless there is a reason night-time behaviour is observed, such as sharing with a sibling, a friend staying for a sleep-over, or during an illness.

Does it tend to get better anyway?

Development of the problem in those for whom it begins early in life has not previously been described and the natural history is currently unclear.

What can be done to treat it?

Four medications have shown reasonable evidence of benefit: melatonin, clonazepam, pramipexole and paroxetine (however the published studies are only on adults and none with ASD).

In addition, a range of other conventional medications (acetylcholinesterase inhibitors, benzodiazepines, carbamazepine, clozapine, desipramine, L-DOPA and sodium oxybate) and one Chinese herbal formula (Yi-Gan San) have all been reported to be of benefit in smaller numbers of cases.

- *Melatonin* has produced improvements in the symptoms of RSBD in over 81%, based on data from 38 cases in four published adult studies.

- *Clonazepam* produced improvements in RSBD in over 91%, based on data from 339 cases in 22 adult trials.

- *Pramipexole*, a dopamine agonist, produced improvements in over 80%, based on data on 29 cases across three trials, all in adults. The results across trials are variable.

- *Paroxetine* was specifically used in one trial with RSBD because it has been shown to reduce REM sleep. This trial reported some success in 16 of 19 cases. In addition, there are single case reports of both benefit and deterioration. It is a selective serotonin reuptake inhibitor (SSRI), a class of medications that have generally been found to make RSBD worse rather than better.

In general, medications that increase serotonergic activity should be used cautiously because this can increase movement during REM sleep.

How likely is it to respond to treatment?
No trials on treatment of RSBD in children or in ASD have been published.

The family doctor referred Tom to the sleep clinic at the local paediatric hospital. They recommended an overnight study of his EEG and breathing and an appointment was made for him to come in overnight the following Friday.

After the admission Tom and his family had it explained to them that his unusual night-time behaviour was a condition called REM sleep behaviour disorder and that this results in him moving and acting out his dreams where other people stay still in this stage of sleep.

This clarified what Tom's problem was, but what could they do to help? The treatment research they could find had been limited to date, and most of the published work is with adults. After discussion, and having the various treatment options explained to them, the family felt that a trial of melatonin was the first strategy Tom might try (although not the most successful treatment reported to date, it has a history of use in children and adolescents including those with ASD, is well tolerated and has no significant side-effects).

Tom started on a course of melatonin he was prescribed through the clinic and his parents found that they didn't hear him up at night as often. He seemed to be sleeping more soundly and couldn't remember his dreams with any detail when asked – previously his descriptions had been graphic and detailed.

He is going to go in for a further overnight sleep study but so far his problem seems to have resolved.

IN A NUTSHELL

A variety of medications and one Chinese herbal treatment have been reported to have shown some success, most in only a small number of cases. As there are no treatment trials, it is impossible to compare their effects or say how likely any is to produce improvements.

No treatments so far have been trialled in children or in ASD.

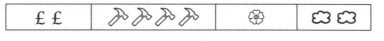

8.4 SHORT NIGHT-TIME SLEEP (HYPOSOMNIA)

— 'Why doesn't she sleep?'

Fiona, who is 16 years old, has never seemed to need much sleep. She is a large girl for her age and is preoccupied with her weight and dieting. Her parents were exhausted with her as a baby, when they were lucky if she would sleep briefly for 20 minutes before waking and demanding attention. When she was 9, because of concerns about her lack of friends and her level of social anxiety she was referred for assessment and diagnosed with Asperger syndrome.

Her sleep pattern has improved in that she will now sleep for six hours, more or less, without a break, but this continues to be far less than other girls of her age.

She is revising for her exams and is becoming increasingly worried that she will perform poorly because of her sleeping difficulties. She tends to sleep more poorly when she is anxious. Her family see academic success as one way in which Fiona can compensate for her social difficulties and feel at a loss over how best to try to help her.

What is hyposomnia?

Short night-time sleep (hyposomnia) is where there is a significant lack of sleep – the person affected regularly sleeps less than normal.

Hyposomnia and insomnia differ. In insomnia, the sleep pattern is often broken and the problem is identified from the presence of persistent difficulties. In hyposomnia, the sleep *pattern* is normal, without more frequent night-time waking, but the amount of time asleep is shorter.

Definition is relative to normal for a given population and is a statistical difference. Many individuals need noticeably less sleep than others and do not want or need help, although it may trouble people they sleep with.

One study reports on sudden adult-onset hyposomnia beginning after a road traffic accident caused by damage to the brainstem in a 32-year-old Caucasian man. He made a good recovery from his accident, but developed chronic hyposomnia. He reported that now he only needed around two or three hours of sleep, compared with sleeping 7.5–8.5 hours before the accident. He did not see himself as having a problem and was pleased at his new alertness and energy, however his wife complained about being disturbed by this new pattern (Guilleminault, Cathala and Castaigne 1973).

How common is it?

In rare cases, hyposomnia begins with a trauma. Defined statistically, we could say that hyposomnia affects 2.14% of the population. Various studies have looked at sleep duration and found differences by age, sex and the population studied.

Poor infant sleep is a risk factor for becoming overweight in childhood. An American study, Project Viva, looked for any links between sleep pattern at 6 months, 1 and 2 years and the children's body proportions at 3 years. Children reported to sleep for less than 12 hours per day in infancy were more than twice as likely to be overweight at 3 years than those who slept for longer (Taveras *et al.* 2008). A typical 6-month-old infant sleeps for around 14.5 hours, but a normal pattern can be anything between 11 and 17.5 hours (see: Iglowstein *et al.* 2003).

Does it tend to get better anyway?

This is a difficult question to answer, as there is no good longitudinal data. There will always be a bottom 2.14% of the population. What we do not know at this point is whether this is the same 2.14% at different ages – is a short sleeper in infancy always going to sleep for less time than others as they get older?

What can be done to treat it?

In one 31-year-old man with severe developmental disabilities, being sleep deprived seemed to escalate aggression (O'Reilly 1995). He used his aggressive behaviour to escape from uncomfortable social situations. Restricted sleep seemed to increase aggressive episodes – the two behaviours seemed to be mutually reinforcing. Reducing social demands reduced his aggression and his sleep improved. Both improvements were maintained over seven-month follow-up.

A 'faded bedtime with response cost protocol' was used to treat sleep problems in two girls (aged 3 and 19) and two boys (aged 4 and 13), referred with self-injurious behaviour, learning difficulties and insomnia (Piazza and Fisher 1991). Each was given a set bedtime close to their typical bedtime, which was gradually made 30 minutes earlier each night. If they were not asleep within 15 minutes of the time set, they were kept awake for one hour, then the whole process was repeated. All four showed improvement which was maintained at follow-up.

How likely is it to respond to treatment?

There is insufficient evidence to tell. Very few papers have reported on this issue, all on small numbers, with no controls. All that can be said is that the treatments used to date have been feasible, acceptable and seem to show clinical benefits.

— Fiona and her parents agreed that they would try a 'faded bedtime with response cost protocol' for her difficulties. They discovered that her 'sleep hygiene' was poor – she would revise in her bedroom until far later than was sensible, and would relax on her bed playing music on her headphones or watching her TV for breaks.

A first step was setting a clear study routine, using a table in the dining room, with breaks as before, but not in her room, and a fixed bedtime which was gradually moved forwards by half an hour each night if she had been successful the previous night until she reached her target. Success was linked to a reward scheme, building towards her earning riding lessons when they went on holiday after her exams.

By the end of the first week, Fiona was getting to bed two hours earlier, and sleeping for eight hours a night. She was surprised that she was actually getting through her revision better than before and school was more pleased with her progress.

IN A NUTSHELL

Functional analysis and tailored behavioural intervention based on this has resulted in improvement in a number of published cases. The types of programme used would probably require some professional help to use, but could be implemented at home and have no significant risks attached. No proper trials have been conducted and only small numbers have been reported, so it is not possible to say *how* likely treatment is to work, only that there is evidence that it has helped in some cases.

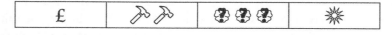

£			

— 9 —

PROBLEMS DURING SLEEP

The Common Parasomnias of ASD

9.1 NIGHTMARES

Exit, pursued by a bear.

(stage direction for Antigonus in William Shakespeare,
The Winter's Tale, Act 3, Scene III)

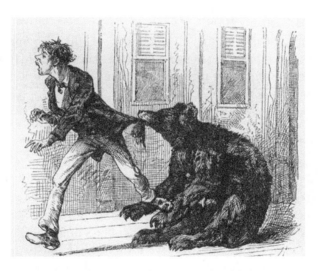

Source: from Mark Twain's Life on the Mississippi, *1883*

━ Charlotte, who is 4, has recently been diagnosed with 'high-functioning autism'. She is a bright girl who achieved all of her developmental milestones and the tests given to her by her paediatrician indicate she has precocious but unusually rigid use of language. She has had to move nursery three times because of complaints from other parents about her behaviour towards their children, and her parents, who both work, are worried that they are running out of local options.

In recent months she has started to wake everyone in the house by screaming hysterically and inconsolably in the middle of the night.

When her parents go into her room to see to her, she is usually awake and talks about what has frightened her – something which she usually describes as being chased through a dark forest by a bear and running to escape from it.

What are nightmares?

Nightmares are typically defined as recurring episodes in which the person affected wakens from sleep able to recall dream content that they find intensely disturbing. This usually involves feelings of fear or anxiety, but may include other dysphoric emotions such as anger, sadness and disgust. The sufferer is generally fully alert on waking immediately after a nightmare, and appears to have intact recall of their dream experience. Settling to sleep can be delayed after such episodes (see: American Academy of Sleep Medicine 2005, 2014). Nightmares seem to happen primarily on waking from REM sleep (Hasler and Germain 2009).

In many people with ASD, because of their communication difficulties, nightmares can often be difficult to discriminate from other conditions causing night-time distress, like night terrors, nocturnal seizures and REM sleep behaviour disorder.

How common are they?

There are few studies on the prevalence of nightmares. One study suggested that bad dreams/nightmares affect around 13.5% of nursery school-age children (Muris *et al.* 2000), and another that nightmares affect some 41% of 6–10-year-olds (Salzarulo and Chevalier 1983).

The first prospective study of preschool bad dreams collected data on 1434 Canadian infants who were followed from 29 months to 6 years (Simard *et al.* 2008). Maternally reported rates were lower than predicted, with the percentage of children being reported as 'often or always having bad dreams' being between 1.5 and 4.2%, peaking at around 3.5 years.

Nightmares are more commonly reported in females than males at all ages (see, e.g.: Nielsen, Stenstrom and Levin 2006).

Retrospective assessments of frequency are unreliable, so it is important to collect a prospective baseline before thinking about intervention (see: Lancee, Spoormaker, Peterse and van den Bout 2008). You need to see how often they actually happen, not how often you think they might have.

Do they tend to get better anyway?

Although nightmares seem to be most common at around 3.5 years, many with bad dreams at 2 are still in the same pattern at 6, so for most the problem is quite stable. Nightmares that begin early seem most likely to persist, while those that start at around 2–3 years, a particularly active period of brain development, seem more likely to improve spontaneously.

What can be done to treat them?

The current treatment of choice is CBT, particularly using a technique known as 'imagery rehearsal' (see: Spoormaker and Montgomery 2008). This is only likely to be effective in someone with ASD who has reasonable language and metacognition (the ability to share thoughts, feelings and ideas).

Imagery rehearsal (Marks 1978) is a method where the person who experienced the nightmare records it in detail, substituting a new ending to the story. This technique can be used individually and has also shown some success as a self-help treatment (Burgess, Marks and Gill 1994).

There is a strong evidence base for imagery rehearsal, however the only direct comparison to exposure/desensitisation found no differences in outcome (Kellner *et al.* 1991).

One early study (Graziano and Mooney 1982) provided 2.5–3-year follow-up data on the use of three weeks of relaxation training as a self-control strategy for night-time fears. 39 out of the 40 children originally enrolled in the study were rated as improved at the end of the three weeks; 31 out of 34 families reported maintained improvement.

Another early study used relaxation exercises, reinforcement and cognitive self-instruction with six children who had severe night-time fears – 5 out of 6 significantly improved (Friedman and Ollendick 1989). In this study, however, improvements were reported before the treatment had begun so may indicate something else, like reduced anxiety, was helping.

Other approaches with supportive evidence are exposure/ desensitisation and the medication prazosin.

Most work so far has been with adults whose nightmares began after trauma and is largely from one research group.

Only one study so far (Krakow *et al.* 2001) has used imagery rehearsal with younger subjects, in the treatment of nightmares in adolescent girls. Most of these girls' nightmares appeared related to sexual assault or abuse. At baseline the 9 treatment and 10 control girls had around 20 nightmares each month. Imagery rehearsal produced a 71% drop, with no change in frequency in the controls. A three-session programme was used. The first session covered information on how nightmares can affect sleep. In the second, they were taught the use of imagery and seven additional techniques: thought stopping, breathing, grounding, talking, writing, acknowledging and choosing. In the third session they learned a three-step process: 'select a nightmare', 'change it any way you wish', and using imagery rehearsal for that dream. They were encouraged at first to write down their nightmares and new dreams, and to move on to doing this mentally if they felt confident to.

Imagery rehearsal has been used to treat both chronic and acute-onset nightmares resulting from trauma from combat and from sexual assault (Krakow *et al.* 2001).

A similar approach, called 'dream reorganisation' was successfully used in treating a 10-year-old boy (Palace and Johnston 1989). This used systematic desensitisation to the dream content with progressive relaxation to keep calm, coupled with practising thinking through the dream to a positive ending.

Lancee, Spoormaker, Krakow and van den Bout (2008) carried out a systematic review of the research on CBT treatments for nightmares. They identified nine RCTs described in 12 papers. Both exposure and imagery rehearsal produced benefits, but the quality of the research was variable and further research was recommended.

Relaxation training alone has shown some success in treating nightmares, but was less effective than desensitisation in 32 adults with chronic nightmares who were randomly allocated to the two approaches (Miller and DiPilato 1983).

Treatment of other sleep problems such as sleep-disordered breathing can often resolve nightmares without any direct focus on treatment of the nightmares themselves (Krakow *et al.* 2000).

Prazosin is a blood pressure-lowering medication with some evidence of benefit. Three small studies describe its use in treating nightmares. It is a maintenance treatment and nightmares return when medication stops. Other medications have had poor or inconclusive results.

How likely are they to respond to treatment?

There is limited published evidence on the treatment of nightmares in children and none on their treatment in ASD. Imagery rehearsal, desensitisation, relaxation and prazosin all have some evidence to support their use. Evidence is mainly on the treatment of acute onset nightmares that were triggered by trauma.

The outcome results so far obtained on PTSD-related nightmares are promising but may be found to differ from results with the more typical chronic idiopathic nightmares seen in childhood.

— Charlotte's parents recently went to their doctor to discuss her nightmares and to see if there was anything that could be done. She explained that this is a fairly common problem at this age and she is likely to improve over time. She was not optimistic about a role for medication, but referred Charlotte for further tests at their request – an overnight EEG with oxygen saturation – but neither showed up anything significant.

A baseline sleep diary showed that Charlotte woke screaming a fairly predictable period of time after going to sleep – never less than 90 minutes and no more than three hours. She was settled in bed usually by 8pm and, on the nights that they occurred, sometime between 9.30 and 11pm a nightmare would begin.

Her parents decided, in consultation with a behavioural psychologist, to try an approach that involved three components:

1. Charlotte learned a simple form of relaxation training which could help her parents to calm her when she was distressed.

2. They would gently waken her at 9.30, re-settle her, reading a story if she wanted it, to 'reset her sleep cycle'.

3. Together with Charlotte, they chose a wallchart with flower stickers for nightmare-free nights (Charlotte had roughly four episodes per week on baseline).

They discussed 'imaginal desensitisation'. They decided that this would be difficult to carry out reliably at Charlotte's age, but planned to try it if the relaxation, re-settling and reward programme did not work.

After six weeks, Charlotte's nightmares had reduced to fewer than one a week and they all decided that no further help was needed over this.

IN A NUTSHELL

There is a limited evidence base showing benefits from imagery rehearsal, systematic desensitisation, relaxation training and prazosin, but the literature is almost exclusively on nightmares secondary to acute trauma.

Imagery rehearsal, systematic desensitisation and relaxation training:

£	🔨🔨	❁❁	☀

Prazosin:

£	🔨	❁❁	☁

9.2 NIGHT TERRORS

▬ 'He just seems to wake up, scream and scream and scream.'

Simon, who is 5, often wakes his parents by moving around his room at night; his parents usually hear him moving around a couple of hours after he has been put to bed. If they go through, he will normally be crying loudly or screaming, and appears to be frightened and very resistant to cuddles or reassurance. He is usually sitting up at the end of his bed, flushed and sweating.

He resists physical contact, pushing anyone away who tries to settle him. He usually appears distant, as if he is still half asleep. Often he will quiet down and return to sleep after a few minutes.

Simon's parents have been told that this is a normal phase and he will grow out of it but find these episodes difficult to understand and are worried that he may be having seizures or that there is something else wrong with him that has been missed.

What are night terrors?

Night terrors (*pavor nocturnes*) are parasomnias in which the person wakes from slow-wave non-REM sleep usually highly upset. In night terrors the person is distressed but unable to give a reason for this, unlike nightmares in which they can usually describe a frightening dream.

Sometimes night-time distress is epileptic in origin (Lombroso 2000), but most is not.

How common are they?

Night terrors are most common between 2 and 6 years of age, when approximately 15% of children are reported to have such episodes.

Do they tend to get better anyway?

One large survey found 2.2% of adults continued to have night terrors (Ohayon, Guilleminault and Priest 1999). Given the prevalence in preschoolers it looks as if around 85% can be expected to improve. What is unclear is the time course and how many cases will persist through childhood and adolescence.

One study looked at night terrors in 161 identical and 229 non-identical twin pairs at 18 and 30 months (Nguyen et al. 2008). At 18 months, 36.9% fulfilled criteria for night terrors and at 30 months 19.7%. This shown a 50% drop over a fairly short period, however the reported rates at both times were extremely high.

What can be done to treat them?

Medication

In a number of early studies, benzodiazepine medications such as midazolam were shown to suppress Stage 3 sleep and reduce night terrors (Fisher et al. 1973; Popoviciu and Corfariu 1983). Midazolam seemed well tolerated, eliminating night terrors in the majority and improved patient-reported sleep quality.

Jan et al. (2004) reported on the treatment of night terrors and sleepwalking in a 12-year-old boy with Asperger syndrome. Therapy involved the use of melatonin to correct sleep-phase onset delay and resulted in the resolution of both problems within two days of beginning treatment.

Waking and re-settling

An early paper (Lask 1988), reported on treatment of 19 children aged 5–13 referred for sleep terrors without comorbid problems. After keeping a baseline record, parents were asked to rouse the child 10–15 minutes before they typically woke. In all cases, the problem resolved within a week of starting this routine. In three cases the problem came back but improved again using the same approach.

How likely are they to respond to treatment?

Night terrors are a common problem in preschoolers that tend to resolve spontaneously in most cases. The limited published data shows that management by night-waking and re-settling, benzodiazepines or melatonin, have all been successful in resolving persistent night terrors. To date, however, the evidence base is small and no RCTs have been reported.

The waking and re-settling approach advocated by Lask is minimally invasive, has no obvious side-effects and could be used with all ability levels, so would seem a sensible initial strategy.

— Simon's parents decided to monitor the pattern of his night terrors for a fortnight before deciding what to try. After keeping a baseline diary, they discovered that his pattern was regular – the episodes were most nights and roughly two hours after he got into a sound sleep.

Simon chose a book to have read to him and they decided that they would read to him for a few minutes if he was difficult to re-settle. In the event, waking him gently around 90 minutes after getting to sleep, and settling him back down rarely got him fully awake and he could usually be settled back to sleep within five minutes.

After a week of rousing and re-settling him, during which he woke once, two hours after he was re-settled, Simon's night terrors subsided completely.

IN A NUTSHELL

A limited evidence base exists for all of the approaches reported to date: night-waking and re-settling, benzodiazepines and melatonin.

| £ | 🔨🔨🔨 | ✿✿✿ | ✳ |

9.3 BEDWETTING (NIGHT-TIME ENURESIS)

Happy is he who gets to know the reasons for things.

Virgil (70–90 BCE), Roman poet

▬ 'His bed is always saturated and he refuses to wear anything at night. We're sure he does it just to annoy us.'

Roberto is a 9-year-old boy who has a diagnosis of ASD. He has additional motor problems and a diagnosis of 'Becker-type' muscular dystrophy. He attends a school for children with moderate learning problems.

He shares a room with his 6-year-old younger brother, Tony. Tony has recently started teasing him about being 'smelly' and being a big boy who still 'pees his bed'. Tony's teasing began not long after he became dry at night about a year ago, and he resents not being allowed to have friends for sleep-overs – his parents are uncomfortable about other families finding out about Roberto's wetting.

Roberto's parents Dave and Diana had made a big fuss over Tony becoming dry and hoped this would encourage his brother. If anything he became resentful of Tony and tried to boss him around whenever he had the opportunity. Roberto is now fully continent during the day but is self-conscious about his problem at night and won't sleep-over with other children if they invite him or have friends to stay. The problem is made more difficult as he refuses to wear a pad at night and the bedding is usually soaking. The family regularly replace his bedding and he has had to have a number of replacement mattresses. This has placed additional financial strain on the family.

The family normally go on camping holidays because they do not want to risk the embarrassment of being asked to leave a resort or hotel. They have not been on a foreign holiday since Roberto was 5.

Although he appears to relate well to his peers in school, his parents are worried that he is getting progressively more isolated outside as the issues around his night-time wetting continue and they feel he could get teased about it or get bullied.

The family have recently approached their doctor for help and have been referred to an 'enuresis clinic' at the local paediatric hospital.

What is enuresis?

Enuresis is the term used for losing voluntary bladder control and passing urine. Night-time (or 'nocturnal') enuresis is where the person wets themselves during sleep – urinating in their nappy (diaper)/

incontinence pad, or wetting the bed. People who bedwet are typically dry when awake, but if they have both bedwetting and daytime accidents this is called 'diurnal' enuresis.

There is nothing to suggest that nocturnal enuresis is deliberate but it can often seem to be and can be a source of stress between children and parents. Where it persists, it can often cause the child to become self-conscious, being reluctant to accept invitations to sleep-over at friends, to invite friends to sleep-over, or to go on school trips that involve overnight stays. Any form of incontinence can lead to teasing and stigmatisation by peers and it is not uncommon for children to move schools because of these 'secondary problems'.

There is evidence that children who bedwet and have never been dry may have immaturities in the key brain structures involved in the control of urination (Lei *et al.* 2012). So in some cases bedwetting may be less easy to control due to slower development of the brain structures involved.

How common is it?

The majority of children are dry through the night by the time they enter full-time education. There is no 'normal' pattern and there is a wide range of individual variation both between individuals in the same population and across cultures.

The typical definition of night-time enuresis is that someone wets their bed twice or more a week. In childhood, the rates of nocturnal enuresis remain fairly high but gradually reduce with age, at age 5 affecting around 15%, with around 15% of them improving each year. Problems are approximately twice as common in boys than girls.

The ALSPAC study followed a large group of children born in southwest England. By 7.5 years, approximately 15.5% of children still had some degree of night-time wetting, 1% were wet most nights and 0.2% wet once or more nightly (Butler *et al.* 2005). This last group, and children who are still wetting regularly by age 10, are unlikely to improve without help.

Does it tend to get better anyway?

In an Italian study of adolescents with persistent nocturnal enuresis, 22% had failed to respond to medication (desmopressin), 23% had had poor compliance to any therapies offered when they were younger, while 40% had not been offered any form of therapy (Nappo *et al.* 2002). In 80% of the cases they reported the problem was severe. 60% were males, most (82%) had a family history of bedwetting, and most (74%) were primary enuretics – they had never had a period of good night-time control.

Children with night-time-only wetting tend to respond more successfully to treatment than children with day-time and night-time difficulties (Fielding 1980).

A study of 2109 women examined current and childhood urinary symptoms (Fitzgerald *et al.* 2006). Eight per cent reported childhood bedwetting and 10% reported nocturia (the need to urinate frequently at night-time). Childhood bedwetting predicted adult urge incontinence, and childhood nocturia tended to persist into adult life.

Further research is required on the proportion of childhood enuretics that persist. For those that do persist, their problems tend to be severe, and can have major psychosocial consequences.

What can be done to treat it?

There is a huge number of different recommended treatments (see, e.g.: Lyon and Schnall 2010; Wright 2008). To make it easier to go through the various approaches that are available, we will cover these in three sections:

1. behavioural interventions

2. medications

3. alternative and complementary treatments.

1. Behavioural interventions

Two major reviews of the results of behavioural interventions cover simple behavioural and physical approaches (Glazener and Evans 2004), and more complex interventions (Glazener, Evans and Peto 2004).

The review of simple behavioural treatments covered approaches like reward charts, fluid restriction and regular waking and lifting. Thirteen studies were found and in general these approaches were better than no intervention but not as effective as either enuresis alarms or medication. There is an advantage to trying these types of intervention first despite their lower success rate: they are less demanding to use, have a reasonable chance of working and have no significant side-effects.

REWARD CHARTS

These are usually wall charts with stars, stickers or other physical symbols put on by, or with, the person each time they achieve a target. With bedwetting, this will be for something like having had a dry bed, a drier bed than on the previous night or whatever other related goal has been agreed. Usually the chart rewards will be linked to something more tangible like going swimming for having five stickers on the chart within a week.

FLUID RESTRICTION

Parents often restrict night-time drinks on the basis that this will mean the child is less likely to have a full bladder and to wet.

REGULAR WAKING AND LIFTING

This tries to prevent wetting by ensuring that they never have an overfull bladder. This approach tries to get the person to go to the toilet during the night before the bladder is overfull and any accidents occur.

In reviewing more complex behavioural treatment interventions, Glazener, Evans and Peto (2004) identified 18 trials in which a multi-component intervention was used, typically involving dry bed training coupled with an enuresis alarm. The evidence base was insufficient to draw any firm conclusion concerning additional benefit, but there was some evidence for a reduced level of relapse after stopping use of an alarm when both approaches had been used.

RETENTION CONTROL TRAINING (RCTR) ('STREAM INTERRUPTION', 'START-STOP' AND 'BLADDER DRILL TRAINING')

RCTr has shown success in improving the amount of urine that can be retained. Medications such as oxybutynin also have this effect. One early controlled trial of RCTr showed an increase in bladder capacity in 18 enuretic children but sadly there was no improvement in their bed-wetting (Harris and Purohit 1977). In a small proportion of cases improvements in capacity and awareness do resolve enuresis, normally by enabling the child to recognise when they need to wake and use the toilet at night (see: De Wachter *et al.* 2002).

If you want to try this approach, use a reward chart, using a simple reward like a sticker or star for achieving a target and gradually increasing the goal – this could be starting and stopping or time from feeling the need to go.

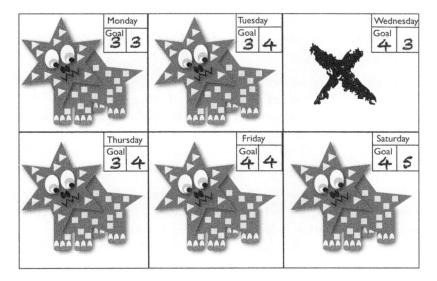

Figure B3: Peter's start-stop shapeosaurus chart

Comparison of RCTr to the use of an enuresis alarm either separately or in combination suggests that both singly and in combination the enuresis alarm contributes significantly more to the management outcome and has a greater chance of working.

DRY BED TRAINING (DBT)

DBT (Bollard and Nettlebeck 1982) is an approach in which, after an initial baseline to establish the pattern of wetting, there is a period of regular waking and toileting, timed to ensure that the child is likely to have a dry bed. Once this pattern has been established, the time between lifts is gradually extended until the child is able to stay dry throughout the night.

This is a very demanding approach for those carrying out the programme, and should not be tried unless it can be properly implemented. This can often require an in-patient admission for the early stages or families to arrange the time to carry out a home-based programme during holidays or over a long weekend break.

ENURESIS ALARMS

There have been many clinical trials of enuresis alarms (the 'bell and pad') (see: Glazener, Evans and Peto 2005). It has the best evidence of any biofeedback treatment for a sleep-related problem, with sustained benefits from treatment.

The approach was first described by Mowrer and Mowrer in 1938. They suggested:

> if some arrangement could be provided so that the sleeping child would be awakened just after the onset of urination, and only at that time, the resulting association of bladder distension and response of awakening and inhibiting further urination should provide precisely the form of training which would seem to be most specifically appropriate. (p.445)

The principle is the same for the alarms used today. By wetting the bed, or, with some devices, a strip worn fitted inside pants, the child's urine completes an electrical circuit setting off an alarm that wakes them.

The point is for the child to associate wetting with being woken and subsequently learning to either wake and go to the toilet or hold on.

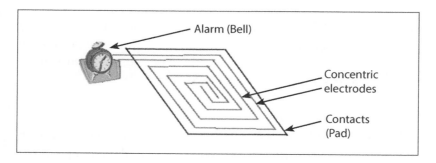

Figure B4: A diagram of the 'bell and pad'

With 14 dry nights as success, in studies comparing use of an alarm to no treatment (14 studies), the alarm was successful in 68% of cases compared to 4% of controls. Alarms are more successful than tricyclic medication, with a lower relapse rate. There is no additional benefit to using both (see: Kiddoo 2007).

The enuresis alarm can work quickly and well in ASD. A recent example established improvement in a 12-year-old autistic girl with foetal alcohol syndrome within three weeks (Henriksen and Peterson 2013).

Alarms that wake the child seem to work best. There is no difference in outcome between those alarms fitted to the bed and those that are worn (usually in modified pants/nappies).

Compared to other behavioural treatments, alarms are more effective in reducing wet nights but no better overall than stream interruption ('stop-start') or dry bed training. Alarm treatment alone is as effective as the combined use of an alarm plus other behavioural interventions.

Alarms have caused electrical burns to children who slept through them (see: Hursthouse 1973). This problem should not happen with any of the current systems.

A list of alarms and where these can be obtained is provided in the Resources section.

2. Medications

Two types of medication, tricyclics and desmopressin, have been used.

TRICYCLICS

A variety of tricyclic medications, such as imipramine, have been prescribed extensively, despite evidence of limited improvement on medication and relapse when stopped. Trials have been reported on imipramine, amitriptyline, viloxazine, nortriptyline, clomipramine and desipramine.

Tricyclic medications contain bioactive compounds that enhance the function of neurotransmitters including serotonin, dopamine and noradrenalin.

Minor side-effects are common, including low blood pressure, dry mouth, constipation, increased perspiration, increased heart rate and insomnia. In addition, overdose can cause heart and liver damage (see: Glazener, Evans and Peto 2003a).

DESMOPRESSIN ACETATE (DDAVP)

Desmopressin works more quickly than an alarm, but improvements are less likely to be sustained, and paradoxically combined desmopressin plus alarm treatment has a poorer outcome than either alone.

DDAVP mimics the hormone vasopressin and reduces urine production. Wetting is reduced because less urine is produced and the bladder does not get distended during sleep.

One study compared DDAVP to oxybutinin or the combination in 114 primary childhood night-time and daytime enuretics and found over 70% improved on DDAVP or the combination while just over 50% improved on oxybutinin alone (Caione *et al.* 1997).

Glazener and Evans (2002) reviewed the treatment literature on children, concluding that it is not a long-term treatment, only improving wetting on the nights that it is used.

DDAVP can cause problems if fluid intake is not restricted. Enuresis alarm treatments are slower to work but have a lower relapse rate. Alloussi *et al.* (2010) reviewed all published studies and concluded that the evidence for DDAVP is stronger in the management of enuresis where there are no other issues and that structured withdrawal improved outcome and lowered the chances of relapse.

Two reviews of DDAVP safety (Van de Walle, Stockner, Raes and Nørgaard 2007; Van de Walle, Van Herzeele and Raes 2010) concluded that the overall safety profile is good. Both highlighted concerns about low sodium levels in body fluids, largely in the elderly. It was suggested this could be an issue at younger ages if high doses were used with inadequate fluid restriction.

OTHER MEDICATIONS

Many medications have been evaluated as possible treatments, the best known being oxybutinin chloride.

A small RCT found that pseudoephedrine (N=11) was significantly better than either oxybutinin (N=9) or indomethacin (N=9) in the treatment of night-time enuresis and that oxybutinin had the highest level of reported side-effects (Varan *et al.* 1996).

The combination of imipramine and oxybutinin was effective and well tolerated in a consecutive open-case-series of 77 childhood eneuretic cases (Tahmaz *et al.* 2000).

The wide range of alternative pharmacotherapies that have been used for night-time enuresis has been extensively reviewed (see: Glazener, Evans and Peto 2003b).

3. Alternative and complementary treatments

A Cochrane review (Glazener, Evans and Cheuk 2005) drew the following conclusions:

HYPNOSIS

There has only been one report on the use of hypnosis to treat childhood enuresis (Edwards and van der Spuy 1985). It was said to produce a better outcome than waiting-list controls. Numbers were too small to draw any strong conclusions and the severity of wetting at baseline differed between the groups.

CHIROPRACTICS

Two small studies support the use of chiropractic treatment for nocturnal enuresis (Leboeuf et al. 1991; Reed et al. 1994). These were inadequate to draw any clear conclusions.

DIETARY INTERVENTIONS

These can be indicated in specific conditions – a low calcium diet has been reported to help some children with enuresis resulting from hypercalcuria (see: Valenti et al. 2002).

Occasionally, bedwetting can be linked to consumption of an enuretic. The dandelion, which in French is appropriately called the 'pis-en-lit' (in parts of Hampshire on the English south coast it is still called the 'pee-the-bed') is one example. In children who engage in pica (swallowing inedible things), unintended ingestion should be checked and excluded and would only be likely if enuretic plants were in season. If found, the remedy is obvious (preventing the person from eating them).

HERBAL REMEDIES

The Chinese remedy *Yi Niao Ling Fang* has been reported as an effective treatment for childhood nocturnal enuresis (Yu-lian, Xiao-yun and Chun-hua 2002) after a study of 96 children aged 5–13 referred for night-time enuresis with nightly wetting. Fifty were treated with *Yi*

Niao Ling Fang and compared against 46 treated with imipramine: 98% of those on *Yi Niao Ling Fang* improved, compared to 73% on imipramine and improvement was maintained at two years. Group allocation and the extent of follow-up for initial non-responders were unclear.

How likely is it to respond to treatment?

Night-time enuresis can be successfully treated in most cases. Mild night-time enuresis (when there are wet beds on fewer than three nights per week) should improve without any intervention, while chronic nightly enuresis is unlikely to resolve without specific treatment (Wright 2008). Spontaneous improvement is unlikely with nightly wetting particularly if it persists after age 10 (Yeung *et al.* 2006). Intervention is particularly important if wetting is chronic (has lasted for several months) and frequent (there are more than two wetting episodes in a typical week).

A small group appear to gain little from clinical treatment. These treatment-resistant cases are typically males with long-standing primary nocturnal enuresis (see: Nappo *et al.* 2002).

Before being referred to the clinic, Roberto's parents thought that bedwetting was rare in boys of his age and that it wasn't connected to his muscle condition. They had been surprised to find that both of these assumptions were wrong. Boys of 9 are still quite likely to bedwet, and this is even more likely in boys who have a condition like Becker muscular dystrophy. As he had become dry by day, and his muscle weakness was mild, Roberto was told that he has a good chance of becoming dry at night. This seemed to change his attitude, now that he thought he could get better, and he has been happier at home and warmer and more tolerant with his younger brother who hasn't been teasing him so much.

The family have been given a buzzer alarm. The sensors were small metal strips that have to be worn in a small pad Roberto secured inside a pair of pants. This is the first time that he has agreed to wearing a pad at night. He has also been taught 'stream-interruption' exercises to do at home and he is keeping a chart of both to take back to the clinic review. To start with progress has been gradual, but he has had two dry nights for the first time ever and is really pleased with himself.

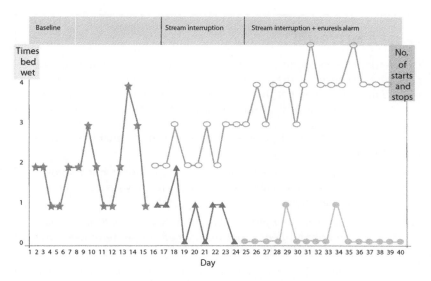

Figure B5: Roberto's chart

IN A NUTSHELL

Wetting the bed occasionally is quite a common problem and is not a cause for concern. If the problem has been persistent for some time, or the person is older than 10, however, it is unlikely to improve without treatment. The following advice applies to these more persistent types of wetting.

Only two types of medication have shown reasonable evidence of benefit:

- *Tricyclics:* These have some reported benefit but improvement is not maintained and there are fairly frequent reports of side-effects.

- *Desmopressin acetate (DDAVP):* This helps over 70% but again the improvement is not maintained, longer term use is not possible and side-effects are quite common.

- *Simple behavioural interventions* (reward charts, fluid restriction, lifting) are often the easiest approach to use initially, but have shown less direct evidence of benefit. Retention control training (RCTr) can be more useful when someone wets often during the night and may have a smaller than average bladder capacity.

- *Dry bed training (DBT)* is a demanding approach but one with some evidence of success in difficult cases.

- *Enuresis alarms:* These have better evidence of long-term benefit than most other approaches. They are best as part of a programme that also uses behavioural intervention to maintain benefits.

- *Alternative and complementary treatments:* There is limited evidence on benefits from hypnosis or chiropractics. Dietary intervention can help in some less typical presentations.

- *Chinese herbal treatments* may have some benefit but there is only one adequate study.

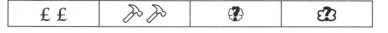

9.4 Sleepwalking (Somnambulism)/ Sleeptalking (Somnliloquy)/ Sleep Groaning (Catathrenia)

▬ **'We often pass him in the hall on our way to bed, walking around the house but fast asleep and oblivious to anything we say.'**

From as early as his parents, Tim and Barbara, could remember, Simon, an 11-year-old boy with ASD, had been getting out of bed quite regularly, several times a week, and walking around the house at night. One time that they did wake him he was confused and anxious, not knowing why he was fully dressed and standing in the hallway. His father, older brother Derek and his Uncle Peter have all gone through periods of sleepwalking, and his father remembers this happening to him again around the time of Simon's diagnosis.

What are sleepwalking, sleeptalking and sleep groaning?

Lady Macbeth sleepwalks in Shakespeare's 'Scottish play' (see: Janowitz 2000); Angel Clare sleepwalks in Thomas Hardy's *Tess of the d'Urbervilles* and Heidi sleepwalks in Johanna Spyri's book of the same name. In all of these fictional examples, it is attributed to some form of stress and a result of worrying external events. There is indeed a link between sleepwalking behaviours and behaviours the person has recently learned while awake (see: Oudiette *et al.* 2011).

In the current classifications, sleepwalking is a parasomnia like night terrors – both seem to happen at the time we change from non-REM sleep (Szelenberger, Niemcewicz and Dabrowska 2005).

'Sleeptalking' (somniloquy) occurs during either sleepwalking, rhythmic movement disorder or bedwetting. The person is typically confused on waking (Nevéus *et al.* 2001).

'Sleep groaning' (catathrenia) is also reported but its nature is unclear. When reported in someone with good normal waking speech, it sometimes appears related to disordered breathing and typically improves when breathing improves (Guilleminault, Hagen and Khaja 2008). In someone who has not developed speech, sleep groaning may be the equivalent to sleeptalking.

How common are they?

Sleepwalking is relatively common in children, and tends to lessen or disappear with age. In a large follow-up study, sleepwalking in childhood was reported in around 26%, dropping to around 3% in adults (Hublin *et al.* 1997). For most children sleepwalking resolves without help.

A number of things are linked to sleepwalking: ADHD (Walters *et al.* 2008), migraine headache (Casez, Dananchet and Besson 2005) and overactive thyroid (Ailouni *et al.* 2005).

Sleepwalking can be a side-effect from medication including quetiapine, olanzapine (Chiu, Chen and Shen 2008) and zolpidem (Hoque and Chesson 2009). It can be associated with restless legs syndrome (see section 8.3.i) or obstructive sleep apnoea (see section 10.4).

In non-identical twins the chances of both twins sleepwalking is around 10–15%. In identical twins, this increases to around 50% (Tafti, Mauret and Dauvilliers 2005). If a parent or sibling sleepwalks the chances in a child are around 45% and if both parents are affected it rises to around 60% (Lavie, Pillar and Malhotra 2005). These associations suggest genetic transmission.

One study has shown a specific genetic basis (Licis *et al.* 2011). Evidence of autosomal dominant transmission (where it could be passed on by either parent), was shown over four generations in one family. All those affected had differences in the 20q12-q13.12 region on chromosome 20 which codes for some 20 functional genes.

Do they tend to get better anyway?

In a study of 33–60-year-old adult twins, out of 1472 pairs, 9.7% of the women and 7.7% of the men reported sleepwalking in childhood. As adults, 3.1% of women and 3.9% of men reported continuing to sleepwalk, but only 0.6% of either sex began to sleepwalk as adults. The majority of those sleepwalking as children do not do so as adults, and adult-onset sleepwalking is extremely rare.

Sleeptalking and sleep groaning are rarer and only seen in a subset of those who sleepwalk. They seem to be part of the general presentation of sleepwalking, but it is unclear if they are indications of likely severity or persistence.

Spontaneous remission is often reported for sleepwalking without any specific type of help.

What can be done to treat them?

Successful psychological treatment was described in two adults whose sleepwalking recurred after stressful events (bereavement in one case and emotional conflict with a sibling in the other) (Conway *et al.* 2011). Coping strategies for dealing with the daytime stressors were used.

A detailed review of the literature on treatment in adults failed to identify an adequate evidence base for best-practice recommendations (Harris and Grunstein 2009).

How likely are they to respond to treatment?

In most cases sleepwalking improves without any need for specific help or a management approach being needed.

In cases where sleepwalking occurs in the presence of RLS or OSA, their treatment will typically resolve the sleepwalking. This is also true where the comorbidity is with ADHD, migraine or untreated hyperthyroidism.

With the sudden onset of sleepwalking after starting a new medication, the possibility that these are associated should be explored. If onset is after a stressful life event, counselling around this event might help.

— Tim and Barbara looked through the literature on sleepwalking. From talking to Tim's parents they also realised that Tim and his brother had regularly sleepwalked until they were in their early teens, as had Simon's brother Derek. In all of them, their sleepwalking subsided with age and the only later recurrence had tended to be short-lived and when under stress. Simon was not worried by his nocturnal wanderings and had never gone out of the house or hurt himself.

They discussed things with the family doctor and, after ruling out migraine, thyroid issues and sleep apnoea, they decided to adopt a 'wait and see' strategy, and sure enough, at around the same age as his brother Simon's sleepwalking gradually faded away until, when they were reviewing things just before his 12th birthday, the family were struggling to remember when it had last happened.

> ## IN A NUTSHELL
>
> Typically things improve when nothing is done and no treatment approach has been shown to be of specific benefit.
>
> Make sure there is no other sleep issue and the problem is not due to a recent change in medication.
>
>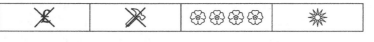

9.5 EXCESSIVE DAYTIME SLEEPINESS/ TIREDNESS (EDS/HYPERSOMNIA)

━ 'He just seems to be tired all the time no matter what we do.'

Sean is a 9-year-old boy who attends a school for children with complex learning problems and ASD. Sometimes he just seems to tire, curls up and naps in class. His teachers find him difficult to wake and afterwards his concentration is poor. His parents have had numerous letters sent home because of his extreme tiredness in school. They have been asked to try to get him to bed early and keep him from doing things that are overly energetic out of school.

They feel the school staff don't believe that he sleeps well at night. Jim and Petra, Sean's parents, have the same difficulties as school with his sleep at weekends and in school holidays. They are worried that there could be something physically wrong with him, and have asked their doctor to refer him for investigation.

What is excessive daytime sleepiness?

Excessive daytime sleepiness (daytime 'hypersomnia') has only been recognised in the past decade. Its causes and its prevalence have only recently come to attention (Mignot 2008).

Excessive daytime sleepiness (EDS) or tiredness (EDT) is essentially a strong, excessive and abnormal daytime compulsion to sleep. It results in an inability to stay awake and alert during the day with unintended lapses into drowsiness or sleep. Diagnosis requires this pattern to be present on most days for at least three months.

Links have been made between EDS and clock gene abnormalities:

- Orexin2-hypocretin2 gene receptor mutations have been reported in EDS with comorbid Tourette syndrome (Thompson *et al.* 2004).

- Low hypocretin-1 levels are found in patients with excessive daytime sleepiness in association with myotonic dystrophy (Martinez-Rodriguez *et al.* 2003). Myotonic dystrophy is associated with ASD. In other cases of excessive daytime sleepiness in ASD this has been in association with hypocretin-2.

In narcolepsy (section 10.5), there is a more complex presentation that can include EDS, cataplexy, hypnagogic hallucinations, sleep paralysis and disturbed night-time sleep.

Various factors predict EDS in adults. One study (Bixler *et al.* 2005) linked depression, body mass index, age, sleep duration, diabetes, smoking and sleep apnoea to EDS (in decreasing order of association). In this sample, rates of EDS reduced with age, as did depression. In men lack of regular exercise, depression and obesity are all associated with higher EDS risk, while in women the major predictor appears to be poorer apnoea-hypopnea scores (Basta *et al.* 2008).

One of the best measures for assessment of daytime sleepiness is the Epworth Sleepiness Scale (ESS) (see: Johns 1991). The ESS can be used in adolescence. Currently the best equivalent for assessment in children is the Pediatric Daytime Sleepiness Scale (PDSS) (Drake *et al.* 2003). This scale is a 13-item self-report measure that has been standardised on a mainstream school sample of 11–15-year-olds in Ohio.

It is helpful to discuss the results of standardised assessments with a clinician familiar with their use. A number of assessments are available to monitor EDS (see: Weaver 2001). Many Internet resources provide copies of scales such as the Epworth Sleepiness Scale, but often with limited information (see: Avidian and Chervin 2002).

How common is it?

EDS is common in adolescents, with almost a quarter scoring at the extreme end of the Epworth Sleepiness Scale and around 14% judging themselves to be extremely sleepy during school hours (Gibson *et al.* 2006).

There is limited data on adults. One early US study reported a rate of 3.4% in 7954 adults (Ford and Kamerow 1989).

In a screening assessment of 2612 adults, increased risk of EDS (based on an Epworth Sleepiness Scale Score of more than 10) was reported in association with ulcers (reported in 9.3%), migraine (16%) and depression (16%) (Stroe *et al.* 2010). EDS was more common the more complex the clinical picture.

There is clearly a need for more systematic epidemiological research to establish how common EDS is at different ages.

Does it tend to get better anyway?

There is no good longitudinal data.

Most adult studies suggest that EDS affects around 5%. If the Canadian figure of 14% in adolescence is replicable in other populations, this suggests that around two-thirds of people who have EDS in their school years improve. There is no useful prospective data on this issue.

Variations in the criteria used and the limited epidemiological data, particularly the lack of longitudinal data, make it impossible to give a clear picture of prognosis (see, for discussion: Ohayon 2008).

What can be done to treat it?

It is helpful to get a confirmed diagnosis and a clear baseline before commencing on any intervention.

Various methods are available to assess the child with EDS. Two measures, the Pediatric Daytime Sleepiness Scale (PDSS) (Drake *et al.* 2003) and the BEARS (see: Owens and Dalzell 2005) can be useful.

A number of strategies can be helpful: improvement to sleep hygiene, treatment of sleep-disordered breathing, the use of bright-light therapy to reset the circadian rhythm, and wake-promoting medications are of particular benefit.

One paper described a programme for 'Robert', a 13-year-old boy with EDS, ASD and learning difficulties (Friedman and Luiselli 2008). Three strategies were used.

1. Stimuli related to sleeping were removed (a soft floor mat and beanbag chair on which he usually slept in school were removed).

2. When staff observed behaviour that usually led to sleep, he was redirected into other types of activity.

3. He was consistently praised for joining in.

This programme stopped Robert's daytime sleeping and was maintained over six-month follow-up.

A number of medications have been used including psychostimulants, modafinil, sodium oxybate, tricyclic antidepressants and SSRIs. A review of EDS medication can be found in Banerjee, Vitiello and Grunstein (2004). Psychostimulants have been most commonly used.

Modafinil use has been increasing, with fewer side-effects than psychostimulants, and lower addiction risk. It improves daytime alertness in adult EDS and appears safe and well tolerated in children. In 10 children with narcolepsy and 3 with idiopathic hypersomnia followed up for 15.6 months, benefits were reported in 90% (Ivanenko, Tauman and Gozal 2003). In the two children with pre-existing conditions (seizures and psychotic symptoms), these worsened.

EDS is commonly reported in Prader-Willi syndrome (PWS) (see, e.g.: Wagner and Berry 2007). PWS is also seen in ASD population (see: Aitken 2010b, Chapter 61). Unlike the other sleep issues in PWS, weight reduction does not seem to help EDS. A preliminary report on three cases suggests modafinil can improve EDS in PWS (Heussler *et al.* 2008).

How likely is it to respond to treatment?

Montgomery and Dunne (2007) were unable to find evidence of any specific treatment trials for EDS.

A useful supportive review on the potential role of modafinil, discussing its use with daytime sleepiness appeared in 2008 (Schwartz 2008).

Changes to the regulation of modafinil introduced by the European Medicines Agency in 2010 currently restrict its use across Europe, including the UK, to those diagnosed with obstructive sleep apnoea (see section 10.4).

━ Philip's family were concerned by his excessive sleeping, and were prepared to try anything to help him become more alert. They were convinced that if this improved his learning would accelerate.

An initial sleep hygiene assessment identified several places and times where he was more likely to start sleeping both at school and at home, typically when he was alone at break times at school or in the living room watching TV at home at weekends. The school agreed to give him a one-to-one auxiliary for a three-week trial to see if this could help to keep him more focused. At home Jim and Petra have started taking it in turns to work with him in the afternoons and don't leave him watching TV when they have things to do at home.

His paediatrician has suggested a trial of stimulant medication. The family are considering whether to try this but are concerned about possible side-effects.

So far the improvements in Philip's daytime alertness have been sustained, he seems to be more interested in school – previously he often objected to getting on the school transport in the mornings, and his school have not sent any recent letters home and Petra is worried about any possible side-effects from longer-term use of medication.

IN A NUTSHELL

There are no well-validated treatment approaches, but two-thirds of those affected in childhood and adolescence will get better without treatment. There is a small literature on successful behavioural treatments and on the use of an alertness promoting medication (modafinil). The use of modafinil has recently been restricted.

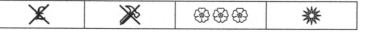

— 10 —

LESS FREQUENT SLEEP ISSUES SEEN IN ASD

10.1 EXCESSIVE NIGHT-TIME SLEEP

━ **'Sometimes we start to think he'll never wake up.'**

Thomas is 11 years old. When he was 6, shortly after making a fairly difficult start to his school career he was assessed and diagnosed as having PDD-NOS (Pervasive Developmental Disorder – Not Otherwise Specified). Ever since they can remember, Thomas has slept for longer than anyone else in the family – as a baby he often slept continuously for 14 hours at a time and his parents were convinced there was something seriously wrong with him. He was getting teased in school for having to be woken up during lessons and often lost his temper and got into fights during breaks when the others pretended to copy him. The family have nicknamed him 'Rip van Winkle' because he is always first to bed and first to sleep at night, but is the last to wake in the morning.

He has undergone various investigations but so far nothing physical has shown up that could account for his excessive sleep and the family have always been reassured that there is nothing physically wrong with him.

What is excessive night-time sleep?

Excessive night-time sleep (nocturnal 'hypersomnia') can be defined as typically sleeping for significantly longer than would be normal for someone the same age.

The best-known condition causing hypersomnia that has so far been linked to ASD is a rare genetic disorder called Kleine-Levin syndrome (KLS). It is caused by an abnormality on the short arm of chromosome 6 that to date has only been described in around 300 people. A subgroup of girls with KLS appears to have cyclical sleep problems linked to their menstrual period (Billiard, Guilleminault and

Dement 1975). KLS is a rare cause of hypersomnia. As hypersomnia is fairly common and KLS is rare, it is an unlikely combination – so far only four people with KLS and ASD – two with autistic disorder and two with Asperger syndrome, have been reported (see: Aitken 2010a).

Hypersomnia does not usually have a known genetic cause. When it results from environmental factors like traumatic brain injury it is called PTH (post-traumatic hypersomnia). This seems to result from damage to the ascending reticular activating system (ARAS), part of the brain controlling the sleep–wake cycle.

Most hypersomnias have no known biological basis. It may be that these cases are just the upper tail of the normal distribution of normal sleep.

How common is it?

Sleep is only excessive compared to what is normal for any given age, sex and population. Excess is a statistical phenomenon rather than an absolute. On this basis it can be said to affect 2.14%.

Around 0.3% have a sleep pattern that would qualify for a diagnosis of 'idiopathic hypersomnia' (Ohayon 2008). It is thought to be underdiagnosed in adults (Vernet and Arnulf 2009).

Does it tend to get better anyway?

As children get older, their sleep gradually settles and typically follows the pattern seen in the area where they grow up. As they get older, they also tend to sleep less.

What can be done to treat it?

Most successful treatments for hypersomnia increase wakefulness and improve attention. Stimulants such as methylphenidate and some other medications with less certain ways of working, like modafinil, have been used. In adults, both approaches seem reasonably successful. One review found improvement or remission in 90% on methylphenidate and 88% on modafinil (Ali *et al.* 2009).

In a study of sleep disorders after traumatic brain injury, one of the two cases of post-traumatic hypersomnia improved with modafinil (Castriotta *et al.* 2009).

In the UK, the use of modafinil is currently restricted to people with a clinical diagnosis of obstructive sleep apnoea (section 10.4).

How likely is it to respond to treatment?

Published clinical studies may only report good responders. Controlled data is required to confirm the results of Ali *et al.* (2009), which suggest success from the use of either methylphenidate or modafinil in most cases.

— After a long discussion with Thomas's physician and after asking everyone else they could think of, his parents felt that there was little else they could do but try a course of medication.

   The doctor recommended a stimulant, and melatonin to get him to sleep at a regular time in case his sleep pattern was too disrupted. He explained that stimulants can slow his physical growth a little and increase his blood pressure but, as he was a big boy compared to his peers already, the effects were likely to be temporary, and his blood pressure (at 100/59) was low normal for his age so no one was too concerned.

   As well as monitoring his sleep pattern the family and school would complete rating scales to measure his activity level, impulsivity and distractability, and he would periodically have his growth and blood pressure checked.

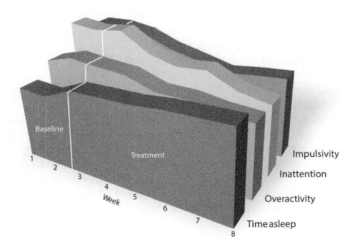

Figure B6: Thomas's sleep pattern

Over eight weeks, Thomas gradually started to sleep for longer and reports both on his progress and his behaviour from school began to improve. He is average height for a boy of his age. There was a slight elevation in his blood pressure (from 104/61 to 111/72), but it remains within the normal range for his age.

IN A NUTSHELL

There is limited evidence but in the published work to date stimulants and modafinil can both be beneficial. These can both have well-recognised side-effects.

£ £	⚒	✿ ✿ ✿	☁

10.2 NIGHT-TIME EATING DISORDERS

'It's as if the eating never stops and we just get ignored when we ask why.'

Julie is an 11-year-old girl with a diagnosis of Asperger syndrome. She has always had a healthy appetite, but over the past 18 months she has steadily increased her snacking at night while watching television with her parents, eating chocolate and biscuits.

Julie's mother Sandra has recently been diagnosed with type-2 diabetes and her father is also overweight. Both Julie's parents are concerned that Julie is turning out to have similar problems and are worried in case she develops diabetes like her mother – they think she would find it very difficult to manage the treatment.

A recent review with the school doctor found that she had gained significantly more weight than expected and she is starting to have difficulties keeping up with her classmates in PE and swimming, both of which she used to enjoy. She is starting to complain about becoming breathless and tries to opt out whenever she can. The doctor mentioned that she might have 'night eating syndrome' (NES), and has made a referral to an eating disorders clinic for further investigations.

Tom is a 13-year-old boy with autistic disorder and learning difficulties. His parents are concerned because they have noticed that he has a habit of getting up during the night and bingeing. This is a pattern that has been noticeable for some months and since starting this he has put on a considerable amount of weight. As there is a family history of cardiac problems his parents worry about the longer-term effects of this pattern on his health if it continues.

A recent clinical assessment resulted in Tom being given a comorbid diagnosis of 'sleep-related eating disorder' or SRED in addition to his autistic disorder and learning difficulties. They did not get any guidance on what they could do to help him but were offered a review appointment for six months. In one way his parents were relieved to be given a diagnosis but became anxious when they could find little information on the condition or on what it could mean for him.

What are night-time eating disorders?

Currently two distinct types of night-time eating problems are recognised – night eating syndrome (NES), and sleep-related eating disorder (SRED).

In NES, the person eats excessively between their main evening meal and bed and/or wakes through the night to eat. People with NES rarely engage in pica (swallowing inedible material). Its onset has not been linked to the use of any specific medication.

From the limited evidence to date NES appears to run in families (Lundgren, Allison and Stunkard 2006). It is commonly associated with mood disorders such as depression (see, e.g.: Vetrugno *et al.* 2006).

Daytime eating disorders are common in people with sleep problems. In an adult series of 60 patients with narcolepsy-cataplexy, 23.3% had an eating disorder, as compared to none of 120 matched controls (Droogleever Fortuyn *et al.* 2008). There is a clinical overlap, with obesity being more likely in someone with NES (Colles, Dixon and O'Brien 2007).

Sleep-related eating disorder (SRED), happens either when fully asleep or when not fully aroused. It involves eating unpalatable or inedible substances (pica) and is associated with a number of other sleep disorders: sleepwalking, RLS and OSA. Onset has been reported after use of hypnotic sedative medication. Zolpidem, triazolam, olanzapine, and risperidone have all been reported as possible triggers (see: Schenck *et al.* 2005).

Where sleep-EEG recordings have been possible, these show SRED happens in an unusual state of arousal and should be classified as a parasomnia, similar to nightmares and sleepwalking.

How common are they?

In adults a prevalence rate of 1.5% for NES has been reported (Striegel-Moore et al. 2005). A population prevalence survey of 6-year old children in a German urban population gave a rate of 1.1% for night-time eating (Lamerz et al. 2005).

There are no published prevalence studies of SRED.

Do they tend to get better anyway?

No studies have followed up people with NES or SRED. The limited cross-sectional information on NES suggests it is more common in adults than children and may be fairly stable over time. There is no data on SRED.

What can be done to treat them?

In NES, sertraline has been reported to help (Stunkard et al. 2006)

As SRED is associated with pica, it is important to check for possible lead toxicity, just as in someone who is awake. Blood-lead levels should be tested in all autistic children with pica (Advisory Committee on Childhood Lead Poisoning Prevention 2000).

A number of medications including dopaminergics, topiramate and benzodiazepines have been reported to help in SRED. Topiramate seems most effective, but has a high rate of side-effects (see: Schenck and Mahowald 2006).

How likely are they to respond to treatment?

One randomised controlled trial of sertraline in NES showed 12 out of 17 cases (71%) improved, compared with 3 out of 17 placebo controls (18%). Other treatments have either not been adequately evaluated at this time (as is the case with non-pharmacological approaches), or shown no improvement.

SRED often improves when other comorbid sleep problems such as RLS or OSA are treated. In cases where the problem is either the only presenting issue or is comorbid with sleepwalking, treatment has so far been largely ineffective (see, for review: Howell, Schenck and Crow 2009).

▬ Julie was seen at the local paediatric clinic and after assessment by both the sleep clinic and hospital dietician she was diagnosed with 'night eating syndrome'.

The family discussed the implications of Julie's diagnosis with the team who made her diagnosis. She has always found taking medication difficult and is reluctant to try sertraline, also saying that she can't see why she has to when her parents eat far more than her.

The family have agreed that they will all go for sessions with the dietician and all try to diet first, and if this does not help Julie they will discuss medication again.

▬ Tom's diagnosis of sleep-related eating disorder concerned his parents, partly because they could find so little information on the condition or on how to treat it. They asked for further investigations – they had noticed that he had begun snoring loudly at night and were also concerned about his rapid weight gain.

Tom's paediatrician has run blood tests for heavy metals and the results showed that he had elevated levels of lead and antimony. The levels were said to be low enough that they would reduce when sources of exposure were found and removed rather than requiring treatment. Several of the surfaces he chewed on proved to have old layers of lead-based paint: an old painted wooden stair-rail and the inside edges of a stair cupboard door. Further tests are being run for metallothionein issues in case he is likely to reaccumulate more rapidly than normal.

The family have been told about various medicines that might be helpful but, as his night-time raids on the kitchen pantry seem to be reducing, they are going to wait until his lead levels are normal before making any decisions.

IN A NUTSHELL

NES and SRED are both recent diagnoses and the literature on them is limited. In both conditions, benefits have been reported from medications as detailed above. If the person also has pica, their lead levels should be checked and treatment for this should be discussed if found to be significantly elevated.

£ £	⚒	✿✿✿	⛆⛆⛆

10.3 Sleep Bruxism (Tooth-Grinding While Asleep)

▬ **'We can hear her through the whole house: it feels like someone is using a road drill in the house next door.'**

Fiona is a 10-year-old girl with autism and communication difficulties. She often appears to be highly anxious and chews at her sleeves if she is told off or gets upset.

When she is asleep, she has a long-standing habit of grinding her teeth together (sleep bruxism). The noise is a high-pitched squeaking sound like fingernails being scraped noisily across a blackboard but can sound even worse from a distance.

Fiona's parents can't remember when she started it but they can't remember her not doing it. The grinding can go on for lengthy periods of 20–30 minutes. Her younger brothers, who have to share the bedroom next to hers, find it difficult to sleep through the noise.

When the bruxism has been particularly noticeable, she often indicates that her jaw is painful the following day.

Although they have looked for a pattern, there doesn't seem to be any link between Fiona's bruxism and any daytime upsets. Grandparents report that both Fiona's father and her paternal uncle had similar night-time problems which resolved when they were in their early teenage years.

What is sleep bruxism?

Sleep bruxism, or tooth-clenching and grinding during sleep is a simple, stereotypic, repetitive and localised sleep-related movement disorder.

How common is it?

Tooth-grinding during sleep typically starts at around 1 year of age, soon after the first incisors erupt. Its prevalence in children ranges from 14% to 20% (Widmalm, Christiansen and Gunn 1995). The reported prevalence by adolescence is around 13% (Strausz *et al.* 2010) and continues to drop, reaching around 3% in old age (Lavigne and Montplaisir 1994).

Bruxism while awake is associated with high stress-sensitivity, anxiety and depression, however there is no evidence to suggest any such link for sleep bruxism (Manfredini and Lobbenzoo 2009), and it is thought that day and night bruxism may represent different conditions with different causes (see: Kato, Dal-Fabbro and Lavigne 2003).

Sleep bruxism is genetic and has shown a significant level of twin concordance (Hublin *et al.* 1998). To date there has been little systematic research to establish the specific genetic or biological basis to this often troubling disorder.

Does it tend to get better anyway?

Fewer people present with bruxism as they get older and there is a reasonable chance that at some stage someone may 'grow out of it'. Adult rates are around 8% and rates in the over 60s some 3%, however, half of all children with bruxism are likely to persist in this habit well into adult life. The only longitudinal study of this phenomenon is a nine-year follow-up of a Finnish population cohort from age 14 to age 23 (Strausz *et al.* 2010). Self-report of tooth-grinding increased in this population from 13.7 to 21.7% over the period from adolescence into young adulthood.

One factor that significantly increases the rate of bruxism is the use of stimulant medications such as methylphenidate, and there is evidence to suggest that the rate of sleep bruxism is increased in stimulant-treated ADHD (see: Gau and Chiang 2009). The chronology is important, therefore, if the onset of the sleep bruxism seems to have coincided with the use of specific medication.

There are a number of case reports of bruxism in association with ASD (Barnoy *et al.* 2009; Muthu and Prathibha 2008).

What can be done to treat it?

A variety of treatment approaches have been advocated including:

- physical devices to prevent tooth-grinding
- transcutaneous electric nerve stimulation (TENS)
- behavioural therapies
- medications.

Recent reviews (Kato and Lavigne 2010; Lang *et al.* 2009) summarise the main treatment approaches.

Physical devices

A range of physical devices has been used to treat sleep bruxism. These include occlusal splints, mouth guards, NTI (nociceptive trigeminal inhibition) splints and mandibular advancement devices (MADs). They have all been studied extensively but there is no definitive evidence of benefit from any. In people with OSA, there is also some evidence that occlusal splinting can interfere with breathing during sleep (Gagnon *et al.* 2004).

TENS (Transcutaneous Electrical Nerve Stimulation)

TENS has been used in one study compared against occlusal splinting (Alvarez-Arenal *et al.* 2002). None of the 11 people in either group experienced pain or headache and the only differences reported were in clicking of the temperomandibular joint on mouth opening and closing which benefited more from splinting.

Behavioural strategies

Two major behavioural strategies have been advocated to date:

1. Lifestyle instruction, relaxation and improved sleep hygiene (where possible minimising the known risk factors for sleep bruxism such as stress, alcohol, smoking and irregular sleep pattern). No outcome studies have looked at the effectiveness of these behavioural strategies alone.

2. Biofeedback, focusing on EMG feedback of tension in the jaw muscles, reduces sleep bruxism, however, as with much other biofeedback fails to show functional carryover once treatment is stopped (Cassisi, McGlynn and Belles 1987; Pierce and Gale 1988).

One study combined CBT with nocturnal biofeedback over three months (Ommerborn *et al.* 2007). Results were no better than occlusal splinting and benefits had disappeared by six-month follow-up.

Pharmacological strategies

To date, only clonidine has shown good results, but with a significant level of reported side-effects.

One paper on the treatment of sleep problems in children with epilepsy found that successful treatment of the epilepsy also produced significant benefit to bruxism in those patients who had exhibited both problems (Elkhayat *et al.* 2010).

How likely is it to respond to treatment?

Currently, there is no well-validated treatment that appears to have a high probability of success without significant side-effects.

Comparisons of the various approaches have concluded that MADs and clonidine have most success. Both are, however, associated with high rates of side-effects, physical discomfort for the MADs and suppression of REM sleep and low morning blood pressure for clonidine.

There is a reasonable spontaneous remission rate, sleep bruxism does not have major problems associated with it and the treatments to date are not without their own problems. Intervention is only really a sensible option if tooth-grinding interferes with other aspects of daily life or relationships.

— Fiona's parents have read everything they could find and looked into the various options.

They have decided that as she has obvious daytime anxiety they will try to use a relaxation and massage approach to make her less agitated.

The night-time tooth-grinding is an issue for the rest of the family but seems only occasionally to cause her jaw discomfort. The various treatments on offer are either effective but with a high rate of side-effects or seem to be of limited efficacy. As there is a reasonable chance that her tooth-grinding will improve in any event, the family have decided not to opt for any form of treatment at present. In the interim they are going to improve the soundproofing in Fiona's bedroom, especially in the wall, floor and roof partition space between Fiona's room and her brother's. This will hopefully make the problem less distressing to the rest of the family, and will let them keep things under review.

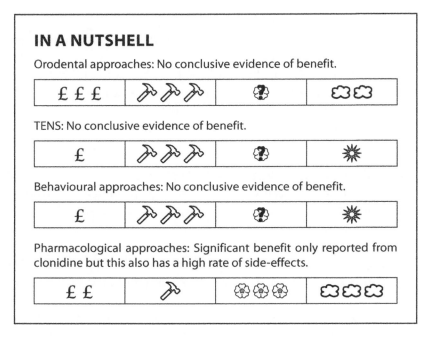

IN A NUTSHELL

Orodental approaches: No conclusive evidence of benefit.

£ £ £	🔨🔨🔨	❓	☁☁

TENS: No conclusive evidence of benefit.

£	🔨🔨🔨	❓	☀

Behavioural approaches: No conclusive evidence of benefit.

£	🔨🔨🔨	❓	☀

Pharmacological approaches: Significant benefit only reported from clonidine but this also has a high rate of side-effects.

£ £	🔨	✿✿✿	☁☁☁

10.4 OBSTRUCTIVE SLEEP APNOEA (OSA)

'He could snore for us in the Olympics.'

Gordon is a 7-year-old boy with ASD who snores loudly in his sleep. When his mother has sat with him at night, sometimes she has also become worried that he often seems to stop breathing for a few seconds at a time. Gordon is overweight for his age and gets easily tired when taking part in sports at school. PE lessons are voluntary and Gordon typically 'opts out'.

He was seen by a clinical geneticist who found that he had a Fragile-X 'CGG expansion', while his mum and one of her sisters have a 'pre-mutational' expansion. His maternal granddad, who is now in his early sixties, has recently developed a hand tremor and is being investigated for something their geneticist called 'FRAXTAS' (fragile-X tremor/ataxia syndrome).

The family are worried that there could be something seriously wrong medically with Gordon and that he could come to harm when his breathing suddenly stops. They have continued to keep a baby sleep-monitor in Gordon's room so that they can hear his breathing. Gordon's snoring is even more intrusive as a result of this and both his parents are now extremely overtired and irritable.

The family recently attended a 'sleep clinic' in the local general hospital and he is being investigated for 'obstructive sleep apnoea'. A first attempt to do an overnight sleep monitor study with Gordon wearing a pulse oximeter, nasal prong and electrocardiogram was a failure as Gordon became distressed at the various leads being attached and stayed awake and upset for most of the night.

What is obstructive sleep apnoea?

OSA is a common form of sleep apnoea (breathing briefly stops with no discernible muscle movement). It is a common paediatric presentation typically linked to being overweight (Katz and D'Ambrosio 2010). Loud snoring is common, interspersed with periods of up to 10 seconds when breathing seems to stop. Raised blood pressure and daytime sleepiness are common.

OSA is more likely to be seen in someone with one of the ASD-related conditions that can result in obesity, such as Biedl-Bardet syndrome, Cohen syndrome, Fragile-X syndrome, Prader-Willi syndrome and Rubinstein-Taybi syndrome (Aitken 2010a).

There is no specific literature on OSA in ASD, and the treatment approach does not differ (see: Gozal 2008).

Untreated OSA often affects daytime cognitive functioning and behaviour (Beebe and Gozal 2002). It can be associated with sleep-disordered breathing, somatic complaints, oppositional and aggressive behaviours and social problems (Zhao *et al.* 2008). Social withdrawal seems to be related more to comorbid obesity, and could interfere with other treatments, so weight-control issues should, where possible, also be addressed (see: Mulvaney *et al.* 2006).

How common is it?

Reported child OSA rates vary between 0.9% and 13% depending on the definition and the data collection method (see: Lumeng and Chervin 2008).

Does it tend to get better anyway?

> *We have begun to understand that sleep disorders in general, and more particularly, sleep-disordered breathing, can lead to substantial morbidities affecting the central nervous system (CNS), the cardiovascular and metabolic systems, and somatic growth, ultimately leading to reduced quality of life.*

(Capdevila *et al.* 2008, p.274)

In children and adolescents with OSA who are overweight, the presentation tends to be worse and the outcome is poorer. Both problems increase risk of adult metabolic syndrome (the combination of insulin resistant diabetes, dyslipidaemia, hypertension and obesity), with the presence of OSA increasing the risk six-fold (Redline *et al.* 2007).

OSA often develops after heart problems or hypertension (see: Smith *et al.* 2002).

What can be done to treat it?

A range of treatments is available (see: Capdevila *et al.* 2008; Halbower, McGinley and Smith 2008).

Treatment of severe OSA might include:

- behavioural intervention

- use of prosthetic devices to maintain an open airway by positioning the jaw or limiting movement of the tongue

- use of mechanical devices to maintain airway pressure during sleep such as CPAP (continuous positive airway pressure)

- in extreme cases that have proven unresponsive to other approaches, surgical intervention (maxillomandibular advancement).

In overweight children, exercise can improve OSA symptoms. In one study of 7–11-year-old children, all improved significantly on the Pediatric Sleep Questionnaire (PSQ) with daily aerobic exercise compared to no additional exercise controls (Davis *et al.* 2006). Improvements in cognitive functioning parallel improvements in aerobic fitness (Davis *et al.* 2007).

Work on behavioural issues may be needed alongside management of OSA in children. Behavioural sleep difficulties present in almost a quarter of children with OSA (22%), the main problem being bedtime refusal. The children with both OSA and behavioural sleep issues are more likely to have daytime behaviour difficulties and daytime sleepiness (Owens *et al.* 1998).

Contrary to popular opinion, most obese people tend to sleep less, not more, than others. Improving sleep hygiene and bedtime routines may be important in OSA-targeted approaches.

Most sufferers have enlarged tonsils and adenoids and improvement in OSA can be achieved in approximately 85% of cases through their surgical removal (Lipton and Gozal 2003).

In the 15% of cases where surgery to remove the tonsils and adenoids is not indicated or has proven unsuccessful, CPAP is the current treatment of choice (see, e.g.: Palombini, Pelayo and Guilleminault 2004). CPAP involves wearing a face mask supplying positive pressure to the face, keeping the airways open during sleep.

Other surgical procedures are used, such as uvulopalato-pharyngoplasty (UPPP or UP3). Most have limited success. The 'Stanford Protocol', however, claims complete cure in 50–70% and significant improvements in a high percentage of all cases (Wietske *et al.* 2007).

Corticosteroid nasal sprays have been reported to have some success in alleviating symptoms (Berlucchi *et al.* 2007).

Orthopaedic devices, worn during sleep to keep the airway open, are reported as being helpful to some (Carvalho *et al.* 2007), but the evidence of significant benefit is disputed (Fox 2007).

For many with OSA, excessive daytime tiredness is a further issue that may also require treatment (see section 9.4).

How likely is it to respond to treatment?

OSA can typically be successfully controlled through one or more of the strategies briefly outlined above. Weight control and improved exercise tolerance should be tried first. If these are ineffective, help may be required through an appropriate paediatric service, and could involve occupational therapy and dietetics.

Differences in definitions and outcome criteria across the studies to date, and the lack of any good medium- to long-term outcome studies make treatment response difficult to gauge. Published studies suggest a high likelihood of improvement or remission when on active treatment, however there is no good longer-term information on compliance or relapse.

Issues such as excessive daytime sleepiness, hyperactivity and inattention can improve when OSA improves (Chervin *et al.* 2006).

In one 5-year-old girl with autism, appropriate treatment of her OSA resulted in an improvement both in daytime behaviour and the severity of her ASD (Malow *et al.* 2006).

— Gordon has the classic signs of obstructive sleep apnoea. The difficulties in overnight recording and his young age both suggested that he was unlikely to tolerate CPAP, where he would need to wear a device overnight to improve his breathing by keeping his airways open. His parents were not keen on his taking regular medication at his age.

As his breathing problem is related to being overweight and could respond to weight loss, the family have decided that they would all exercise more and adopt a healthier diet and lifestyle. They have joined a local gym and now go swimming twice a week as a family.

They are keeping up with the research on treatments for Fragile-X such as the work on mGluR5 blocking agents and hope that some treatments based on this sort of work will soon be available to help Gordon.

IN A NUTSHELL

- *Behavioural intervention:* Often in tandem with other approaches and focused on weight control/exercise tolerance/comorbid sleep issues, not on the OSA directly (rated for these benefits, not effect on OSA).

- *Prosthetic devices:* Various devices, with variable and disputed evidence of benefit.

- *Mechanical devices (e.g. CPAP):* Needs to be worn nightly, improves brain oxygenation but not tolerated by all. Good success rate when used as directed.

- *Medication:* Some limited evidence of corticosteroid benefits but limited research.

- *Surgery:* Other than tonsillectomy, this is a 'treatment approach of last resort'. In extreme cases, the Stanford Protocol has a reported success rate of 50–70%.

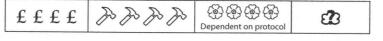

| £ £ £ £ | 🔨🔨🔨🔨 | ✿✿✿✿ Dependent on protocol | 🐛 |

10.5 NARCOLEPSY

— 'Everything is going along fine, then something happens like a balloon popping or a car backfiring and we find him collapsed in a heap on the floor.'

Greig, who is 14, has always had a problem with getting to sleep at night. He will often fall asleep while in the middle of things that hold his friend's interest – at the cinema, on the bus, or while waiting to take his turn when bowling, he often falls suddenly into a deep sleep and is difficult to rouse. He complains that he is a poor sleeper at night, and sometimes that he feels 'stuck to the bed' when he wakes up, as if he is paralysed – he can tell what is happening around him but cannot respond.

Something else his parents are worried by is that he can slump to the ground if he is startled by a sudden noise. This can happen if he hears a car backfire, a starting pistol at a race, or if someone pops a balloon or bursts a crisp packet at a party.

What is narcolepsy?

Narcolepsy has two key features: (1) excessive daytime sleepiness, and (2) sudden loss of muscle tone, usually if laughing or being tickled, but sometimes in response to loud noises or other sudden shocks (cataplexy) (Dahl, Holttum and Trubnick 1994).

It can be called 'Gelineau's syndrome' after the French neurologist who first described it (Gelineau 1880).

There is often disruption to night-time sleep. REM sleep can occur at or near sleep onset and can sometimes result in what are known as hypnagogic hallucinations, a part of the condition, as in Greig's case. There can also be sleep paralysis – when the person feels unable to move when between being asleep and fully awake (see: Cheyne and Girard 2009).

A third of cases begin in childhood, 4.5% before age 5 and 16% before 10 (Challamel et al. 1994).

Assessment and diagnosis typically relies on a multiple sleep latency test (MSLT) – an overnight EEG recording is made, together with recording sleep latency on several daytime naps (Carskadon et al. 1986).

In most cases where brain structure has been studied, the posterior hypothalamus was poorly developed (see, e.g.: Blouin et al. 2005).

A partial loss of hypothalamic cells is seen in 'narcolepsy without cataplexy' (Thannickal, Nienhuis and Siegel 2009) and there is reduced production of the hypocretin orexin (Zeitzer, Nishino and Mignot 2006). Hypocretins are neuropeptides involved in processes that include controlling the sleep–wake cycle (Martynska *et al.* 2005).

Low levels of hypocretin-1 in cerebrospinal fluid (CSF) are seen in 88.5% of cases of narcolepsy with cataplexy (Dauvilliers *et al.* 2003). This could help with clinical assessment in cases where other tests do not provide clear answers (Mignot *et al.* 2002). Obtaining CSF is an invasive procedure, with clinical risks, and should only be done if clearly indicated.

One early-onset narcolepsy case had hypocretin gene mutation (HCRT) on chromosome 17q21 (Peyron *et al.* 2000). A number of other genetic differences have also been reported (4p13-q21; 6p21; 14q11.2; 21q11.2; 21q22.3; and 22q13). Most cases are sporadic.

In 25–31% of identical twins, both are affected, which suggests a strong genetic basis (Mignot 1998).

Cataplexy, when the person loses muscle control, collapsing in response to sudden noise or shock, is almost always seen in people with narcolepsy. It is reported in several rarer conditions associated with ASD, including Coffin-Lowry syndrome and Prader-Willi syndrome (see: Aitken 2010a, 2010b) and in Niemann-Pick type C.

How common is it?

Narcolepsy is rare, affecting around 1 in 2000–5000 people.

Narcoleptic patients may receive a wide range of alternative diagnoses before their diagnosis has been clarified (see: Kryger, Walld and Manfreda 2002).

Does it tend to get better anyway?

It is a lifelong condition but fortunately does not tend to worsen as the person gets older. There is an increased risk of being involved in car accidents, probably as a result of poor attention.

Narcoleptics perform poorly on tests of sustained attention (Findley *et al.* 1995).

What can be done to treat it?

Various treatments have been advocated (see: Aran *et al*. 2010; Kothare and Kaleyias 2008). The general treatment approach typically involves improved sleep hygiene, with daytime naps, and medication.

A range of medications have been suggested:

- Modafinil has been shown to improve alertness in narcoleptics (Littner *et al*. 2001).

- Sodium oxybate has also been found to improve narcoleptic symptoms (Mamelak *et al*. 2004) and reduce daytime sleepiness in narcoleptic patients (Black and Houghton 2006).

- Venlafaxine, an SNRI (serotonin-norepinephrine reuptake inhibitor), has been shown to be of benefit and is the third most used medication currently for paediatric narcolepsy after modafinil and sodium oxybate (Aran *et al*. 2010).

- Methylphenidate, amphetamines and other psychostimulants can be of some benefit (Morgenthaler *et al*. 2007).

- SSRIs have been advocated, but reported benefits are non-specific with a significant rate of side-effects (Nishino and Mignot 1997).

One research letter describes successful treatment of two boys aged 15 and 17 using hypnosis (Weidong *et al*. 2009).

How likely is it to respond to treatment?

The studies published to date suggest that a high proportion of those with narcolepsy can be successfully controlled with modafinil, sodium oxybate or venlafaxine in conjunction with behavioural interventions. Significant improvements are seen in well over two-thirds of cases.

■— After reading the material available over the Internet and discussing with their paediatrician, Greig's parents were reassured that he was not 'unique', and pleased to find that there were a number of treatments that seemed to help, and that they helped most people with Greig's problem.

Modafinil seemed to be the treatment with the best success rate, and they agreed to a trial (after some heart-searching when they found that it did not have a strong record of use in children and there was no clear understanding of why it was supposed to work, and that this would be an 'off label' approach).

Greig started on modafinil (one tablet in the morning and one at lunchtime) and after a fortnight when there had been no 'collapses' they reviewed the recordings they and the school had kept with their paediatrician. The results were unequivocal – he was more alert, participating more and seldom fell asleep. They are continuing with his course of medication and are planning regular reviews to monitor for any issues.

IN A NUTSHELL

There is a small literature as this is a relatively uncommon condition.

From what has been published so far, the appropriate use of medication together with improved sleep hygiene and a behavioural management strategy seems able too improve things in most cases.

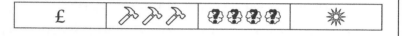

10.6 HOW TO DECIDE IF ALL YOUR HARD WORK HAS BEEN WORTHWHILE

You have spent a lot of time and effort working out what the problem was, and the best course of action to deal with it. It is important to know if it has worked. (Is the problem any better?/Has it improved?/ Has there been an acceptance that the behaviour is within normal limits?)

When things have improved, can you tell what made the difference (e.g. you might have anticipated having to use a complex intervention but found that improving sleep hygiene was enough)?

Sometimes people only feel better about a problem because they have a consistent way of dealing with it (maybe with fewer disagreements and people getting on better and not from improved sleep).

Monitoring reasons for success can be useful – it should help you to remember what you need to do if it comes back; when you need to address other issues; if you need to ask for additional help, it should help to exclude things that are less likely to work and streamline the process.

If you are working through this book systematically, you should have a clear baseline profile of the frequency and severity of the sleep problem that you were trying to alter, have carried out a functional analysis as described above, identified the problem and tried out your solution. This put you in a good position to gauge whether what you did has improved things.

There are essentially six possible outcomes:

1. Complete improvement – the problem has resolved with no ongoing issues.

2. A sufficient change that nothing else needs to be done.

3. Some improvement but a need for further change.

4. No real difference between the problem now and during the baseline recording – the results are inconclusive.

5. Things have got worse.

6. No effect.

These outcomes are displayed in Figure B7 as profiles from eight weeks of hypothetical sleep recording data (from the beginning of January to the end of February) with a rating of 20 at the start of intervention.

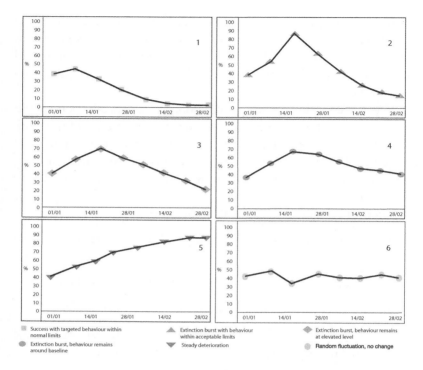

Figure B7: Patterns you might see in your recordings

In the ideal world you will have achieved outcome 1 or 2. The problem is better and you have a clear idea of how to tackle things should any problems recur. If you have achieved outcome 3, the strategy is working but needs to be continued, or the initial intervention may need to be adapted to achieve the desired result. With outcome 4 you will need to try an alternative approach, as your formulation seems to have been incorrect – whatever you changed had no effect. If you have outcome 5, nothing else has changed, and you have given sufficient time for things to improve, you have clearly identified relevant factors that influence the behaviour but not how they are operating – the changes seem to be making the problem worse for longer than would be seen with an 'extinction burst' and you need to see how these influences could be reversed.

The reason for emphasising the need to leave sufficient time is that in some cases there is an extinction burst – the problem can get worse before improving. If, for example, at baseline the child woke, cried out and seemed to find being consoled rewarding, you might have decided to ignore them then, giving more attention when they were settled to bed and in the morning on waking. In the initial stages the problem would probably have increased as the child was unaware that you had changed how you were going to respond.

Maintaining improvements

Having identified the key factors that maintain the sleep problem, changed these and brought about an improvement, it is equally important that you are able to keep these gains.

If the problem was primarily behavioural, letting your programme slip and allowing the problem to build up again could make it more difficult to succeed as quickly if you need to work through the same approach a second time – the child will have learned ways to get around the programme and achieve what they want, and is less likely to respond.

It is important to maintain a watching brief, for the early weeks at least, to ensure that the problem has been successfully dealt with.

Table B2: Summary table: Sleep disorders and treatment choices

Sleep disorder	Treatment of choice	Key evidence	Reported success rate for treatment	Possible issues
Difficulty settling to sleep and frequent night-waking	Behavioural	Multiple studies, see: Ivanenko and Patwari (2009); Moore, Meltzer and Mindell (2008)	70%	None
Insomnia	Behavioural and cognitive-behavioural + medication	Espie and Kyle (2009)	70%+	None
Short night-time sleep	Behavioural	O'Reilly (1995); Piazza and Fisher (1991)	Evidence base too small to compute	None
Excessive night-time sleep	Modafinil	Ali et al. (2009)	88% (1 study only)	Recent restrictions on use
Excessive daytime sleepiness/tiredness	Modafinil	Ivanenko, Tauman and Gozal (2003)	Modest benefits in all (1 small study)	Exacerbation of seizures and psychotic symptoms
Nightmares	Imagery rehearsal; desensitisation; relaxation; prazocin	Krakow et al. (2001); Lancee et al. (2008)	Most studies with traumatic onset nightmares	Lack of maintained improvement with prazocin alone
Night terrors	Night-waking and re-settling; benzodiazepines; melatonin	Jan et al. (2004); Lask (1988); Popoviciu and Corfariu (1983)	High spontaneous resolution rate; no RCTs	Uncertain due to limited evidence base
Night-time eating disorders	Sertraline; topiramate	O'Reardon, Stunkard and Allison (2004); Stunkard et al. (2006)	71%	Topiramate most effective but with a high rate of side-effects

	Medication – type dependent on diagnosis		No reliable data	Dependent on medication of choice
Nocturnal seizures		Bazil (2003)	No reliable data	Dependent on medication of choice
Sleep-related rhythmic movement disorder		Picchietti and Picchietti (2008)	Self-remitting in most cases	No relevant safety data on ropinirole
Sleep bruxism	Orodental; behavioural; clonidine	Huynh et al. (2006); Huynh et al. (2007)	Unclear	MADs can cause physical discomfort; Clonidine can cause REM suppression and low morning BP
Obstructive sleep apnoea	Weight reduction; improved fitness; CPAP	Capdevila et al. (2008); Halbower, McGinley and Smith (2008)	80%+	Discomfort from CPAP and prostheses; general risks from surgery
Narcolepsy	Improved sleep hygiene coupled with medication (modafinil, sodium oxybate, venlafaxine or psychostimulants)	Aran et al. (2010); Kothare and Kaleyias (2008)	70%	SSRIs have significant side-effects but are not first choice for management
Nocturnal enuresis	DDAVP; enuresis alarm; behavioural	Evans (2001); Lyon and Schnall (2010); Wright (2008)	79%	Results with DDAVP do not generalise
REM sleep behaviour disorder	Melatonin; clonazepam; pramipexole; Yi-Gan San	Aurora et al. (2010); Gagnon, Postuma and Montplaisir (2006)	No studies in relevant populations	Variable dependent on treatment of choice, see reviews
Restless legs syndrome and periodic limb movements in sleep	Improved sleep hygiene; iron supplementation	Trenkwalder et al. (2008)	There are no long-term outcome data on RLS or PLMD	As for SMRD: no relevant safety data on ropinirole

PART C

SLEEP

WHAT IS IT AND WHY DO WE DO SO MUCH OF IT?

This part gives a brief summary of our current understanding of sleep.

We evolved on a planet with alternating light and darkness. Unlike some of its other inhabitants, humans don't see well in the dark. In natural lighting conditions our vision is weak for a significant amount of time, every day. It helps to understand sleep if we recognise that it evolved as one way we cope with this repeating pattern generated by the movement of our Earth, its Moon and our Sun. As the Earth rotates on its axis, at any time half the world is bathed in sunlight (cloud-cover permitting) while the other half is in darkness.

Before we learned how to use fire to give warmth and light after the sun set, there was little to do after dark except stay still, keep warm and conserve energy. Sleep was a good survival strategy as it reduced the risk of being killed by predators with better night vision.

WHAT IS SLEEP?

Most of us spend about a third of our lives asleep. Few if any of us understand what it is. Most definitions say little more than that it is a recurring period when we are inactive and unresponsive and that it seems to be good for us.

Our sleep EEG shows periods of REM (rapid eye movement) sleep. During REM sleep, brain activity disconnects from control of our bodies – a bit like like a car being put into neutral – we become motionless and silent. Before we lived in houses this would have made sleeping safer – these days we might fall out of our low beds onto a carpet, but for our ancestors this might have been from somewhere high up and out of easy reach of predators. Minimising movement would have made us quieter, less likely to fall and less likely to draw unwanted attention.

Asleep we are more vulnerable to being eaten, attacked or having an accidents. It seems a risky business, closing down our awareness, making us physically unproductive sitting targets repeatedly, every day of our lives.

Sleep is a surprisingly social activity. Before birth we are affected by changes in our mother's heart rate, her voice and her breathing, and are awash in amniotic fluid rich with her fluctuating hormones and peptides. We react to change in the lights, sounds and movements that envelop us, and learn to recognise the darkness that usually accompanies our mother's sleep. Our own sleep falls in step with our mother's both before and after birth and, after we are born, most of us will rarely sleep alone.

When we sleep together, either with one other person or in a social group, our sleep tends to synchronise, as do other aspects of our biologies. Maternal–infant separation disrupts infant sleep and increases stress. Given how social our natural sleep is, it seems odd that most research continues to treat sleep as a solo activity.

Babies often sleep best when they can hear an adult heartbeat, something that has been constant for them since mid-pregnancy when they began to register sound. In most societies infants continue to co-sleep with their mothers throughout their early life.

Sleep has evolved over recent human history:

- *Changing darkness:* Group recreational activities began to happen more after dark once we could make fire to keep ourselves warm and deter predators. Today's patterns of evening dining, nightclubs, pubs, filmgoing and TV watching mean that more of our lives are now spent awake at times that we evolved to be asleep.

- *Changing diet:* We have changed from being hunters only eating fruit and vegetables in season through finding ways of farming, preserving and transporting foods to today consuming a year-round abundance of a wide range of foods. Rapidly evolving farming methods and novel ways of preparing and preserving food have changed the nutritional make-up of our diets. Today few people hunt, grow, process or even cook their own food.

- *Changing sources of advice:* Historically we relied on the advice of surviving elders in our immediate social group. Today we tend to be swayed by 'professional' advice on childrearing. We are now far more likely to be influenced by the advice of an anonymous agony aunt on television, a media doctor, a book like this one or a web resource.

Other changes have come about through scientific progress:

- the systematic use of fire for heat, light and cooking
- preservation of food by drying, pickling, bottling, canning and refrigeration
- wearing clothes
- artifical light
- written language – with the wider permeation of advice
- central heating
- air conditioning

and, of course:

- the ubiquitous effect of television (see, for discussion: Jenni and O'Connor 2005).

Many modern sleep difficulties come from being able to work and play when we evolved to be asleep (night-time shift work only emerged when we were able to make it bright enough at night for work). Other problems result from technological advances that allow us to move rapidly around the world across timezones (jet lag only arrived with the advent of longer distance passenger aircraft, not with the more sedate pace of the ocean liner or the steam train).

WHY DO WE SLEEP?

We all need to sleep and gear our bodily patterns to the world around us. The 'best guess expert views' on why this happens are not very illuminating:

> If sleep does not serve an absolutely vital function, then it is the biggest mistake the evolutionary process has ever made... (I Allan Rechtschaffen 1978, p.88)

> Sleep remains one of the great mysteries of biomedical science. Few physiologic processes are as fundamental to health and function, so universal in daily experience, and so poorly understood... (Rochelle Tractenberg and Clifford Singer 2007, p.1171)

Our sleep patterns differ due to various factors including stress, exercise, diet and genetics. We are still uncertain about what, if anything, sleep is for, or the effects of variation in our sleep patterns.

In these increasingly obese and weight-obsessed times, it is interesting that if your sleep fluctuates, you are more likely to gain weight. If sleep is restricted this increases both appetite and ghrelin levels but decreases levels of leptin, so having less sleep tends to go hand-in-hand with an increasing waistline.

BIOLOGICAL CLOCKS

'Biological clocks' are cellular mechanisms controlled by 'clock genes' with a regular time pattern. They control variations in body chemistry, temperature and immune function and regulate our sleep patterns. Biologically driven differences in sleep pattern are common in people with ASDs (Glickman 2010), and some come from clock gene differences.

There seems to be a separate process that links tiredness to 'sleep-deprivation'. This helps us compensate for times when we use more energy by taking more sleep.

We all have times of the day when we seem to be at our best. Our thinking ability has a circadian pattern and is affected both by our biological clocks and by external factors affecting our sleep. These differences seems to be real and partly account for variations in performance. Exam scores are affected by the time of day they are taken and how well this matches the person's 'chronotype' (Goldstein et al. 2007).

Some sleep theories

There is no reason to sleep

One theory is that sleep is trivial and just something to do because we are resting (you could think of this as the 'there's nothing decent on the telly' view). This seems like saying that we only have a brain to stop our ears from banging together when we walk.

The opposite view has also been argued: sleep must have an important function because otherwise it would have been selected out by evolution, we just haven't figured out what it is important for.

Against this view is that there are at least some positive and negative consequences: on the plus side, there is selective enhancement of memory and also conservation of energy, on the minus side, our vulnerability while asleep and our reduced ability to do anything else while sleeping.

Sleep enables storage of relevant daytime memories

In animals it has been shown that a small structure deep in the brain (called the hippocampus) increases activity when learning. During subsequent sleep this same area increases activity again and seems to be backing-up and strengthening new memories.

Babies also learn and remember new associations while asleep (Fifer *et al.* 2010).

This is only true for some types of memory, however.

Brief periods of sleep can improve learning and retention but this can easily be disrupted by sleep deprivation.

Sleep is just a by-product of 'other important stuff going on'

Another idea is that sleep might just be part of a system in which changes in the relationships between nerve cells result in the release of certain chemicals, and that sleep is just a 'bystander effect' from this. On this view, we may not need to sleep, but we need to alter our metabolism in a way that ends up with sleep happening as a by-product (this could be called the 'you can't make an omelette without breaking eggs' model of sleep). It overlaps with the first theory above – sleep is not important in itself but happens because of something else important going on.

If this is view is correct and we understood the neurochemistry we might one day be able to promote the chemical changes we need while stopping or reducing the amount of sleep.

Sleep is a way to replenish energy

Sleep could be a way to restore our levels of certain molecules like adenosine and glycogen that are important for brain function and which run down when awake. This 'energy hypothesis of sleep' may apply to a range of circadian metabolic processes.

Some support for this view comes from research showing that brain areas that are more active while an animal is awake show more slow-wave electrical activity during subsequent sleep.

Sleep is just an evolutionary remnant

A different type of view concerns why sleep may have developed during evolution. Sleep may have been important in our history and no longer be required but, because it has no strong disadvantage, has not yet disappeared from human behaviour. On this view, sleep is a remnant of a once important system we no longer require (a 'sleep as an appendix' model). Sadly, if this view is correct there is no way to confirm it. The fact that sleep seems to be a phenomenon seen in all species raises questions – are humans unique in not requiring sleep but for some reason doing it anyway?

Table C1: Theories of sleep

Theory	Support	Against	Key reference
Sleep enables storage of relevant daytime memories	Sleep activates areas used during waking task learning (in mice at least)	Only certain types of memory are enhanced	Hill, Hogan and Karmiloff-Smith (2007)
Sleep is just a by-product of 'other important stuff going on'	No direct supporting evidence – conjecture	Not currently testable	Krueger, Obal and Fang (1999)
Sleep is a way to replenish energy	Various essential compounds such as adenosine and glycogen build-up during sleep and reduce while awake	No contradictory evidence	Benington and Heller (1995); Scharf et al. 2008)
Sleep is just an evolutionary remnant without any real function	No direct supporting evidence – conjecture	Not supported by evidence from any of the above	Rial et al. (2007)

WHY DO WE DREAM?

To sleep, perchance to dream – ay, there's the rub.

(William Shakespeare, *Hamlet*, Act III, Sc. i, 65–68)

For some people, dreams seem to be important and relate in some way to waking experience. Some therapies, particularly psychoanalysis, place great importance on the significance and interpretation of dream content.

During REM sleep, our brains show unique patterns of activity related to recent waking experience. When someone wakes from REM sleep, they tend to remember their dreams, even in children as young as 2. A small proportion of people who wake from non-REM sleep can also remember dreams.

Researchers have suggested that during REM sleep our brains might be involved in reorganising and adjusting emotional aspects of our behaviour, and in modulating and regulating, and even preparing for daytime activities.

Our daytime moods and our sleep patterns interact – poor sleep affects our waking mood and being moody when we are awake causes poor sleep. A number of accounts of dreaming focus on links with emotional and physical health (see, e.g.: Palagini and Rosenlicht 2010).

Theories of dreaming

Threat rehearsal

The sleep researcher Antti Revonsuo (2000) suggests that dreams 'rehearse' how we might deal with threatening situations. He tries to explain the seemingly irrelevant and disturbing content of many dreams. Dreams could be a way of mentally rehearsing different 'what if?' scenarios, some of which might then happen.

There is a rare medical condition known as 'REM sleep behaviour disorder'(RSBD). Those with RSBD physically act out their dreams during sleep (see: Budhiraja 2007). When the dream involves violence, they can hurt themselves or others. This suggests that during dreaming people really can imagine being involved in risky situations. This seems to support the theory, but it can't be the whole story.

Many dreams seem to have no link to potential or past threatening experiences. The relevance of such acting-out dreams must surely also wane, but recurring dreams often seem to be vivid. This pattern does not sit easily with threat rehearsal being our only reason for dreaming.

Virtual reality

For J. Allan Hobson, dreaming is 'protoconsciousness'. REM sleep and dreaming is a hard-wired form of virtual reality when possible scenarios can be imagined as we sleep. This view overlaps with the threat rehearsal model, but for a broader range of possible experiences.

Random activation

The 'random activation' or 'activation-synthesis' theory proposed by Hobson and McCarley (1977) suggested that dreams are a spin-off effect occurring when the brain compares an internal model of how the world works against past experience. On this view, dreaming is a consequence of a particular brain process that occurs during sleep.

Mental decluttering

A different view is that dreaming could be a sort of mental *feng shui*, allowing unwanted associations and memories to be discarded while retaining more useful ones. John Hughlings Jackson is quoted as saying that the role of sleep is to 'sweep the higher layers of the highest centres clean' of unnecessary neuronal connections or memories (see: Taylor 1932). The clearest statement of this theory comes from Frances Crick and Graeme Mitchison who suggest that dreaming occurrs when unwanted neural associations are weakened (Crick and Mitchison 1983).

Memory consolidation

Another view, proposing the opposite, is that dreaming can strengthen recall of new material.

In one study, students learned to play a new video game over a period of three days and were asked to recall any dreams that involved playing the game. The more novel the game seemed to them, the more likely they were to report dreaming about it (Stickgold *et al.* 2000).

Epiphenomena

Dreams may be a by-product or side-effect of some other bodily process. This amounts to saying that there is no reason or purpose for dreaming. We just dream because we do (see, e.g.: Flanagan 2001).

Table C2 shows the main theories suggested as explanations for dreaming and dream content.

Table C2: Theories of dreaming

Theory	Support	Against	Key reference
Threat rehearsal	Dream content links to predicted stressors	Much dream content seems unrelated to expected future events	Revonsuo and Valli (2008)
Virtual reality	No direct supporting evidence – conjecture	Analogy not science	Hobson (2009)
Random activation	No direct supporting evidence – conjecture	Difficult to quantify proportions of content	Hobson and McCarley (1977)
Mental decluttering	No direct supporting evidence – conjecture (at the 'it would be a useful thing for it to do' level)	Evidence suggests differences in consolidation not recall suppression	Crick and Mitchison (1983)
Memory consolidation	Reported dream imagery can reflect recent learning experiences	Consolidation is selective suggesting this is a partial model at best	Stickgold *et al.* (2000)
Selective memory	Emotional events are consolidated by REM, neural memories are not	A partial model at best	Nishida *et al.* (2009)
Epiphenomena	No direct supporting evidence – conjecture	Contradicted by the above	Flanagan (2001)

Sleep may help retain memories of arousing events. This could provide a simple mechanism for selective memory consolidation. As we evolved, we would have benefited most from being able to recall and learn from arousing situations – hunting, escaping predators, procreation and so on. One study supports this idea, reporting that REM sleep strengthens emotional but not neural memories (Nishida *et al.* 2009). The linking of arousal with memory of successful strategies would have actively selected for the survival of people who dreamed about their successes while selecting against people who did not.

A cursory overview of theories of sleep and dreaming shows an overlap (other than the obvious point that we dream when asleep) – both may be important for memory consolidation, both may be evolutionary leftovers and neither may be important for anything. It is clear that we are looking at educated guesswork about what sleep and dreaming achieve, not at any clear understanding.

Sleep and dreaming are slippery philosophical concepts, but it is much easier to study their physical processes: changes in our brain activity, metabolism and body biochemistry while we are sleeping or dreaming. What do we know about them?

WHAT HAPPENS TO US WHILE WE SLEEP?
Electrical brain activity

An EEG records brain activity using electrodes on the surface of the scalp. The numbers of electrode pairs vary, and an overnight recording may use around 20. A computer stores and can play back the recording, usually along with measures of heart rate and respiration and oxygen levels in the bloodstream.

Sleep is currently said to have four 'stages', each with its own EEG features and associated behaviours. Electrical activity also changes with age. Slow-wave activity changes are associated with specific stages in brain development and can be used to trace cortical development.

Blood flow and metabolism are slower during sleep, and differ across sleep phases. Although there is an overall drop in metabolism, the higher-order networks involved in thought continue to operate and interconnect.

When you are awake, an EEG shows variable activity. During sleep, this pattern changes.

Stage 1 sleep

This stage is 'light' sleep, when someone can easily be woken. The person is generally more physically relaxed than when awake, but physical twitches and jerks are commonly seen.

REM sleep

REM is a single sleep stage, but has two phases called 'tonic' and 'phasic' REM. In tonic REM, people may react to external events but in phasic REM they are unreactive, and an fMRI shows a 'functionally isolated thalamocortical loop'. This complex pattern of brain activity seems to provide a clear physical basis to dreaming – almost as if someone was awake, but isolated from the outside world – all of the action is, quite literally, happening inside the person's head.

In adults, REM sleep usually happens after around 90 minutes of sleep but onset is faster when overtired or 'sleep-deprived'. REM is the stage when nightmares typically occur.

Infants and neonates have a 'compressed' sleep cycle and can go rapidly into REM sleep. This is why babies can often happily maintain sleep patterns that completely exhaust their parents.

Most infants sleep for longer overall with a high proportion of time spent in REM. A normal baby can sleep for up to two-thirds of the day spending roughly half of it in REM. Teenagers spends around one-third of their time asleep but only one hour is REM, and an adult will typically spend even less time asleep, of which less than 20% will be in REM. Our sleep pattern changes markedly and predictably as we get older.

Autistic children both take longer to go into and have less REM sleep than others (Buckley *et al.* 2010). Results differ across studies and might reflect the different neurobiologies of the ASDs (Coleman and Gillberg 2011).

Stage 2 sleep

The EEG shows patterns called 'sleep spindles' (also called sensori-motor rhythm or SMR) and 'K complexes'. Muscle activity is reduced and the person seems unaware of events. Sleep spindles seem related to screening out external sounds – the more sleep spindles, the better someone can sleep through noise.

A pattern known as CAP (cyclic alternating pattern) is seen during Stage 2. CAP is often slowed in autism (Miano *et al.* 2007) and Asperger syndrome (Bruni *et al.* 2007), and in other disorders of arousal, in learning difficulties and in ADHD.

Stage 3 sleep

The Stage 3 EEG consists mainly of low frequency (0/5–2 Hertz) slow or delta waves. Many sleep problems are most common during this stage. Night terrors, rhythmic movement disorder, bruxism, nocturnal enuresis (bedwetting), sleepwalking and sleeptalking occur mainly during Stage 3.

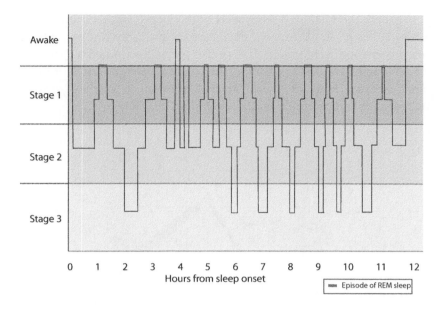

Figure C1: The stages of sleep

Verbal people with ASD are more likely than others to report insomnia or a phase-advanced sleep cycle, often reporting they sleep later (Limoges *et al.* 2005). They can take longer to get to sleep, wake more often and have lower sleep efficiency (the amount of time spent in bed compared to the amount of time asleep).

They spend longer in Stage 1, and have decreased non-REM and slow-wave sleep, fewer sleep spindles and fewer eye movements during REM.

Biochemical changes that happen while we sleep

A number of well-studied chemical changes are also associated with sleep.

Growth hormone

Growth hormone is released in pulses in tandem with melatonin during Stage 3 sleep, when over half our growth hormone is produced.

Excess production is associated with sleep-disordered breathing and implicated in obstructive sleep apnoea, probably through effects on growth and weight gain. It may also play a role in narcolepsy.

A number of ASD conditions involve excessive physical growth, and elevated levels of growth-related hormones including growth hormone binding protein may be seen (Figure C2).

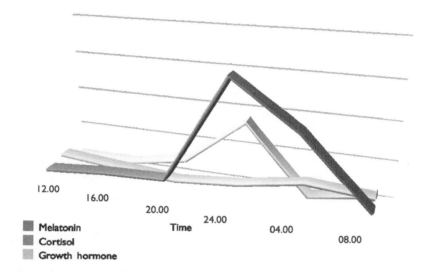

Figure C2: Circadian hormone fluctuations

Cortisol

Cortisol is an adrenal secretion with a circadian rhythm that is affected by sleep and daytime arousal. Boys and girls have similar patterns. The highest levels are found around waking and the lowest in the early stages of sleep.

One study of urinary cortisol levels in 18 high-functioning autistic boys found a normal circadian pattern, with a slight elevation in some (Richdale and Prior 1992). A study on adolescent boys with Asperger syndrome found no elevation of cortisol levels on wakening (Brosnan *et al.* 2009).

Thyroid stimulating hormone

TSH (thyrotropin) is a pituitary hormone involved in controlling the thyroid gland.

It has a clear circadian pattern with the highest levels recorded at night. TSH is produced in distinct pulses with an average of nine pulses over a day, clustering with the highest TSH levels between 2 and 4am. This is paralleled by changes in other biochemical factors affecting thyroid metabolism.

Abnormal TSH levels are seen in a number of sleep problems such as obstructive sleep apnoea, restless legs syndrome, sleepwalking and insomnia.

Melatonin

Melatonin is made from tryptophan, an essential dietary amino acid which is converted to serotonin and then to melatonin.

Low bodyweight and low 'ponderal index' (a measure of the ratio of body weight to length) at birth predict lower melatonin production in adulthood. Both are risk factors for obesity.

Adult melatonin levels show a clear circadian pattern with higher levels before sleep. These gradually reduce through the night and waking occurs typically when they return to daytime levels.

The critical role of melatonin in human circadian rhythm has been used to argue for the use of melatonin supplements or melatonin agonists in the treatment of sleep disorders. Melatonin is currently the only widely used endocrine treatment in the treatment of sleep disorders in ASD.

Adenosine

Adenosine is one of the four ribonucleic acid (RNA) nucleosides. In its free state it also has a number of metabolic functions.

Animal studies show circadian fluctuations in adenosine in a range of body tissues, linked to maintaining energy homeostasis. It is thought to play a role in regulating sleep. Giving adenosine agonists (medications that increase its metabolism) induces sleep while giving antagonists decreases sleep.

Adenosine levels are affected by both caffeine and chocolate intake – increased levels of either suppresses REM. This suggests that taking hot chocolate as a bedtime drink might help people who were troubled by nightmares or other REM sleep conditions, although this could have other less desirable consequences. There is no evidence on the effects of varying adenosine intake on sleep.

Prolactin

Prolactin is produced by the pituitary gland. It is a hormone that stimulates breastmilk production by the mother after birth. Its release has a circadian rhythm with elevated levels during sleep and lower levels on waking.

A number of animal studies have shown that prolactin levels correlate with the overall amount of REM sleep.

Testosterone

Testosterone is produced by men and women but in significantly higher amounts by men. Its circulating levels show a circadian rhythm, with the highest levels typically around 8am and the lowest around 8pm. These patterns are established well before puberty and are reported from 4–5 years of age. Levels are also affected by the level of ambient sunlight.

Testosterone secretion is disrupted by broken sleep, and levels are lowered in conditions like obstructive sleep apnoea.

There is a close correlation between fluctuations in the levels of circulating testosterone and of luteinising hormone. In women, the rapid rise of luteinising hormone, an anterior pituitary hormone, triggers ovulation.

Leptin

Leptin is involved in fat metabolism with higher levels in overweight people. There is a clear chronobiotic pattern in the general population. The highest levels are found at night and the lowest levels around midday. Levels are twice as high in women as they are in men, but fluctuations show a similar pattern.

Leptin levels are directly associated with seizure control and epilepsy. The levels vary inversely with markers of pituitary-adrenal function such as adrenocorticotropic hormone (ACTH).

Elevated levels of plasma leptin have been reported in early-onset autism (Ashwood *et al.* 2008).

Ghrelin

Ghrelin is a peptide found in the hypothalamus and stomach. It is involved in appetite control and promoting sleep. Higher levels are associated with increased slow-wave sleep. Levels vary in a circadian pattern, higher at night-time and lower in the morning.

Abnormalities have been reported in inflammatory bowel disease, epileptic seizures and with immune abnormalities, all of which have been linked to ASD. It has been suggested that ghrelin could be a therapeutic target in the treatment of epilepsy, but to date there has been no published work supporting this.

Insulin

Insulin is a pancreatic hormone that controls blood glucose. Abnormalities can result in diabetes. It is involved in the regulation of the body's carbohydrate and fat metabolism.

Insulin levels vary with sleep stage. In general, lower levels are seen during REM and higher levels during non-REM sleep.

Elevated levels of two insulin growth factors (IGF-1 and IGF-2) and of insulin growth factor binding protein 3 (IGFBP-3) are seen in many with ASDs, accompanied by faster head and body growth.

Glycogen

The body uses glycogen to store carbohydrates, and genes involved in glycogen metabolism are important in circadian rhythms.

When we stay awake for too long, our brain glycogen levels fall and are replenished during sleep. Most brain glycogen is found in support cells called astrocytes. Glucose provides the major source of nervous system energy, with glycogen playing a relatively minor role, however changes in glycogen seem to be a better gauge of brain energy demands.

In addition to these chemical and electrical changes in activity within the brain, there are changes in factors like breathing rate and body temperature.

WHY GOOD SLEEP IS IMPORTANT FOR YOU AND YOUR BRAIN

Disturbed sleep affects the wiring-up of nerve cells, which in turn affects brain growth and function. It interferes with how well the brain processes information and changes. Persistent sleep problems affect both brain development and learning. Even relatively short periods of deprived sleep markedly interfere with someone's abilities (Gujar *et al.* 2010) and their cognitive and emotional functioning (Yoo *et al.* 2007).

There are now many studies showing differences in how brain areas connect up in autism. None of this work has so far taken the effects of sleep into account.

Identifying sleep issues should be a part of the assessment of any behavioural problems. Effective management of sleep problems can enhance learning and improve behaviour.

How our sleep–wake patterns change as we get older

By around the eighth month of pregnancy, circadian rhythms in brain electrical activity can be seen, including sleep patterns, with REM and NREM sleep, and circadian heart rate and temperature patterns (Figure C3).

The baby's own rhythms are entrained through experience of a range of neurochemical, sensory, circadian and ultradian patterns mainly learned through the mother. These impose temporal patterns on key brain areas involved in timekeeping for the rest of its life.

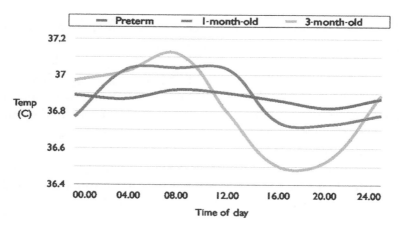

Figure C3: Infant circadian temperature variations
Source: based on material in Glotzbach, Edgar and Ariagno 1995

The infant's progression from unstable to stable sleep

Late in pregnancy, the foetus shows the ability to learn and remember sounds. The sounds heard most will usually be its mother's voice, distorted as it passes both through her body and the amniotic fluid in which the baby floats before reaching the ear. Because of this it will be the patterns not the pitch or tone that the foetus learns. By birth, the infant has already developed a clear preference for the patterns in the mother's voice.

Experiencing other sounds before birth can also lead to recognition and preference. For example, babies who hear specific music during the last three days of pregnancy respond more to this than to other music played to them shortly after birth.

We can improve the social responsiveness of infants who have had less optimal exposure to their mother's voice before birth. Infants born prematurely have missed the period of late exposure before birth, but they could be given recordings of their mothers to help them recognise her patterns; those with congenital deafness and with other sensory issues could also be helped to recognise and respond more to their caregivers.

After birth, there are circadian variations in a host of other things: light levels, the amount of tryptophan, melatonin and SCFAs in mother's breastmilk, the levels and types of ambient sound, and changes in temperature. All help to establish the infant's sleep–wake patterns. It isn't surprising that breast-fed babies generally develop better sleep patterns than bottle-fed ones.

An increased risk of ASD seems to be associated with the use of formula feeds (Schultz et al. 2006), and with prematurity and low birth weight (Limperopoulos et al. 2008). Maternal factors like high blood pressure, type-2 and gestational diabetes also increase ASD risk (Krakowiak et al. 2012).

Early patterning experiences need to be given stronger emphasis during antenatal preparation.

The brain at rest

Our central nervous system is dependent on external sources of energy. Nerve cells lack the mitochondria found in all other cells which produce our main source of energy – a chemical called adenosine triphosphate (ATP). Our brains, therefore, depend on steady supplies of energy delivered by the blood, and from local support cells (called glia and astrocytes). Consequently, neurons rapidly stop working when the heart stops beating and circulating our blood. When cut off from their main energy supply, our brain chemistry rapidly breaks down.

When we are alive, our brains are very difficult things to investigate. We believe that, unlike any other organs, our brains are an essential part of who we are. They are the most critical and delicate part of our anatomy, and the best protected from injury.

The brain researcher faces a host of problems: the brain is encased in bone. As bone is radio-opaque, techniques like X-rays were unhelpful until computer analysis of multiple sources (CAT scanning) let us image the living brain despite the skull. More recently, magnetic resonance imaging (MRI) has given us a system that images water content rather than more dense structures, and does not image bone. This has taken structural imaging to a new level of definition.

Other technologies like EEG; MRI; fMRI, fMRS (functional magnetic resonance spectroscopy), PET (position emission tomography) and SPECT (single proton emission computed tomography) let us look at metabolism, and DTI (diffusion tension imaging) allow us to access aspects of brain function in a way that was impossible until very recently.

There is still very limited systematic data on sleep in ASD but this is a fast-developing area and promises to yield helpful information on brain development, differences and metabolism in ASD and how these are linked (see: Pierce 2011).

SLEEP AND DIET

> Let me have men about me that are fat;
> Sleek-headed men and such as sleep o' nights:
> Yond Cassius has a lean and hungry look;
> He thinks too much: such men are dangerous.

(William Shakespeare, *Julius Caesar*, Act 1 Sc. ii)

Oddly, obese people usually sleep less, not more. This is partly because staying awake longer gives more opportunity to snack. One reason exercise can help with weight loss is that you occupy yourself with things that are difficult to do at the same time as eating.

A range of dietary sensitivities and deficiencies affect behaviour and sleep in ASD (see: Aitken 2008). No dietary factor is critical, but some are particularly important in specific subgroups.

For almost all of us, we began by drinking milk, either from our mothers or prepared infant formula. There are marked circadian rhythms in various components of breast milk including its fat, melatonin, tryptophan and antioxidant content, and in the amount produced. The circadian rhythm of the breast-fed infant's own melatonin production gradually mimics the mother and is established by around 3 months.

Infant formula feeds do not vary in make-up or concentration through the day. The bottle-fed baby gets the same amount, strength and formula of feed day and night. Research shows that parents are more likely to put formula-fed babies into a separate cot or bedroom earlier, cutting off access to sleep cues like parental movement patterns and heartbeat. This combination may account for the significantly higher rates of sleep difficulties found in formula-fed babies.

Infant melatonin levels vary by season of birth, and there are seasonal variations in the birth rate of children with neurodevelopmental problems.

Initiating and continuing with breastfeeding are more likely when mother and infant sleep together (Ball 2003). Breastfeeding encourages a good sleep pattern in the infant, improving immune function, a pattern that would have evolved when this was critical to infant survival.

Adequate intake of tryptophan, an 'essential' amino acid, is another important aspect of diet. It is only available from the diet and cannot be made by the body. It is found in many foods and is the dietary substrate used by our bodies to make melatonin. Bananas, chocolate, oats, dates, milk, yogurt, cottage cheese, red meats, eggs, fish, poultry and a variety of seeds and nuts are rich dietary sources.

As the child gets older, dietary tryptophan intake become more important. One large study of infants and childen found that the amount of tryptophan consumed at breakfast affected both sleep quality and pattern.

Children with ASD are at increased risk of developing epilepsy (see: Canitano 2007). Sleep problems are also more common in this group. The role of lipid metabolism in seizure activity has been shown to be significant in both groups and can respond to change in diet.

One small study of a 'ketogenic diet' was tried with epileptic children not helped by medication. In the children who continued with it, daytime sleepiness reduced, the quality of their sleep improved, and they showed increases in REM. One year later, they still had fewer and less severe fits (see: Hallböök, Lundgren and Rosén 2007).

A few people with ASD have coeliac disease and cannot tolerate dietary gluten. Gluten is found in wheat and some other grains. In general, people with coeliac disease sleep poorly, but this does not usually improve on a gluten-free diet alone.

Some have emphasised the differences in essential fatty acids (EFAs) when comparing breast milk to formula and the possible link with ASD (Brown and Austin 2009). EFA differences are one of many differences between supplemented and unsupplemented formulas. There have been no direct studies of circadian differences in melatonin, tryptophan or of other essential nutrients in ASD.

A wide range of factors alter nutritional effects on sleep, including the action of genes important for the metabolism of cholesterol, amino acids, lipids, glycogen and glucose.

B vitamins play a role in modulating sleep but have had less research attention. Increasing B12 levels can shorten the sleep–wake cycle. As B12, typically in the form of methylcobalamin, has been widely used by families of children with ASD (see: James *et al.* 2009), this approach could cause or worsen pre-existing sleep problems.

Most B vitamins come initially from infant milk, and in breast-fed babies levels are strongly related to maternal diet. In vegans, for example, breast milk is lacking in vitamin B12, which is derived entirely from animal products and cannot be made by the mother's body. B12 is not found in vegetables or fruits.

B12 deficiency due to vegan breastfeeding can cause reversible developmental regression in infants (Casella *et al.* 2005).

Vegan breast milk is also low in taurine, an amino acid derived from cysteine. Cysteine levels are typically low in the vegan diet as it is found at higher levels in animal than vegetable protein.

One three-month randomised controlled trial used vitamin and mineral supplementation in a small group of autistic children with significant parent-reported improvements in sleep and GI issues. Although interesting, the study is too small to draw any useful conclusions, and only three-quarters of children completed the study (Adams and Holloway 2004).

Iron deficiency has been linked to 'restless legs syndrome', and more generally to sleep problems in infancy. Both iron and zinc supplementation can lengthen infant sleep in nutritionally deprived areas (such as Nepal and Zanzibar).

Orexins (hypocretins) are peptides produced in the brain by the hypothalamus. They help to regulate the sleep–wake cycle. Orexin abnormalities have been found in narcolepsy and obstructive sleep apnoea.

REM sleep behaviour disorder has been linked to excessive caffeine (Stolz and Aldrich 1991) and chocolate (Vorona and Ware 2002) consumption.

Alcohol consumption

Eating a large meal can make you drowsy and can be worsened by alcohol. Alcohol can interfere with both arousal and sleep.

If mothers drink alcohol before breastfeeding, this can markedly reduce their infant's activity during sleep, with compensatory increases in motor activity during later sleep. When this happens repeatedly, the infant's sleep pattern becomes poor and unpredictable.

Problems related to alcohol use are not common in childhood, becoming more of an issue in adolescence. Alcohol continues to be the most common drug used by Western adolescents.

The effects of alcohol on sleep and behaviour in adolescence have only recently been studied. There is increasing evidence for an association between substance abuse in general (including of alcohol and tobacco) and adolescent difficulties with sleep, learning and executive functioning.

Clock genes affect our bodies ability to cope with alcohol. Variations in the PER2 gene (2q37.3) have been linked to poorer self-control of alcohol intake. Differences in the PER2 gene have been linked both to excess alcohol consumption and to sleep problems in adolescent boys. Deletions in this gene region have been reported in two studies on ASD (Lukusa *et al.* 2004; Wassink *et al.* 2005).

Diet, genetics and brain development

Our understanding of genetic factors has improved through looking at the effect genes have on appetite and metabolism and the effects that diet has on gene expression

The fact that changes in environmental factors like diet alter how genes work has caused a major rethink in our understanding of genetics (see, e.g.: Francis 2011) and is helping with the development of more effective treatments for sleep disorders (Mignot, Taheri and Nishino 2002).

Diet, nutrient differences and medication can all affect epigenetic processes (see: Junien 2006; McGowan, Meaney and Szyf 2008).

SOCIAL INTERACTION AND SLEEP

Social interaction is also important in the development and regulation of sleep. In the early stages of development, the mother–infant relationship has particularly strong effects on the infant's developing sleep pattern (Donlea and Shaw 2009).

There is a strong association between the presence of sleep problems in those with ASD and parental stress (Doo and Wing 2006), particularly with stress on the mother (Hoffman *et al.* 2008).

Why Mum's laughter is probably one of the best medicines for the growing baby

Laughter is good for you – we may not know why – it doesn't seem to achieve or produce anything, but it feels good. Why do we laugh? Presumably we laugh, chortle, guffaw and giggle for a reason. One reason could be that we find it is difficult to be aggressive when we laugh. Maybe it is a signal that evolved to tell others we feel safe and relaxed.

A roomful of mothers watch a DVD of Charlie Chaplin in *Hard Times*. A second group of mothers watch a similar length DVD (this time of old weather forecasts). After watching the films, both groups breastfeed their babies and provide milk samples over the next 12 hours.

They are all taking part in a study on infant allergic dermatitis, a skin problem which affected their babies. The study was looking at differences in melatonin in the mothers' milk, and whether it was affected by what they saw.

The mothers all report liking *Hard Times*, and typically say they find it funny. None of the mothers are amused by watching weather forecasts. When the milk samples are studied and things put together, the mother's laughter and the levels of melatonin in breast milk are strongly associated – having a fit of the giggles increases breast milk melatonin levels (Kimata 2007). More surprisingly, when mothers breastfeed after watching the Chaplin film their infants' dermatitis improved. One result of maternal amusement seemed to be an improved immune response in her baby.

Laughter boosts immune function (Atsumi *et al.* 2004) and reduces allergic skin reactions (Kimata 2001, 2004). Being happier seems to reduce infection risk and may have evolved to control disease.

Laughter and feeling happy seem to have positive effects, and the opposite is also true – mothers who are depressed and anxious before the birth of their baby (O'Connor *et al.* 2007) and mothers with low mood after the birth (Armitage *et al.* 2009) are more likely to have infants who sleep poorly. Postnatal depression is linked to poorer maternal immune function and more maternal sleep problems.

So far, no one has looked at the other possible associations these studies suggest: Does maternal depression lower breast milk melatonin? Are formula-fed or breast-fed babies of postnatally depressed mothers more likely to show sleep difficulties?

Infants of depressed mothers are less socially responsive, an effect that is stronger for depressive history than for current mood.

Taken together these findings argue for the importance of maternal mood state in establishing and maintaining the infant's developing sleep–wake cycle.

Mother–infant co-sleeping

Infants sleeping with their mother/parents arouses strong opinions. Those against argue that there are increased risks of problems like sudden infant death syndrome (SIDS) from unintentional suffocation (see: McKenna and McDade 2005). This runs contrary to most of the evidence both about the evolutionary development of human sleeping patterns (McKenna *et al.* 1993), and from more recent incidents. If anything, the data suggest that co-sleeping in a normal bed actually reduces SIDS risk. Infant fatalities through co-sleeping typically befall infants whose parents are drug users and involve sleeping prone on a couch or in a high-risk bed such as a waterbed that can more easily restrict infant breathing (McKenna and McDade 2005).

Many children never sleep alone, going from sharing with parent/s to sharing rooms with siblings, and then on to sharing their bed with a partner, often for the rest of their lives. It makes sense to view sleep as a social activity. Co-sleeping is the norm not the exception. As most adults and children co-sleep it seems odd that sleep continues to be studied as a solitary activity.

Infant sleep patterns differ between sleeping alone or with their mothers. Their overall amount of sleep does not differ, but infants who co-sleep waken more often. Co-sleeping leads to more frequent but shorter periods of night-time waking and to faster settling.

Co-sleeping seems to bring the arousal levels of the sleepers into synchrony and may help to alert mothers to infant sleep disturbance and accelerate the maturation of infant sleep patterns by entraining them to their mother.

An early US study of sleep in 6-month–4-year-olds found co-sleeping was typical of 34% of white and 70% of black families. In the white group only, sleeping together became more common as children got older. It was associated with increased stress and lower education and was more common in children who did not fall asleep in their own bed.

Around 1 in 10 babies sleep with their mother/parents in the first year, with a gradual rise in rates through the preschool period, peaking at around 4 years when around 38% of children are reported as co-sleeping once or more every week. At around 4 years more than half spend at least one night a week in their parent's bed. Bed-sharing is not associated with more sleep problems, but the frequency of bed-sharing and night-waking are closely linked.

Not surprisingly, breastfeeding mothers get less sleep when they sleep separately from their babies than do bottle-feeding mothers. In contrast, when they sleep together with their babies, breastfeeding mothers get better sleep than those who are bottle-feeding.

How babies calm themselves

Younger children often 'self-soothe' before sleep. Behaviours like thumb sucking; rolling hair between their fingers; rhythmically body-rocking; or using soothers, teddy bears, dolls and blankets as 'transitional objects' are common. (Favourite objects that are held or stroked can be referred to as 'transitional objects' aiding in the transition from wakefulness to sleep.)

Benjamin Spock, the author of *The Commonsense Book of Baby and Child Care* (1946), wrote that activities like thumb sucking and the use of 'transitional objects' were related. He saw them as mother-substitutes used by children given insufficient access to breastfeeding. He suggested that babies who were breast-fed more regularly were less likely to thumb suck. His work has appeared in a posthumous updated eighth edition (Spock and Needleman 2004).

In reality, there is scant evidence on these issues. Infants who seem poor at self-consoling or at using a transitional object are more likely to develop infant sleep disorders and are more likely to need parental comforting to get to sleep. All infants use some sort of transitional aid getting to sleep, whether an external object, self-consoling or being consoled by a carer. It is not clear how this helps infants to get to sleep, or whether there is anything to be gained or lost through trying to 'break the habit'.

Mary Ainsworth, who pioneered the concept of 'attachment theory', suggested that children who were 'insecurely attached' to their mothers would be more likely to use self-soothing activities. Research has since failed to show any association between attachment and self-soothing or transitional objects.

Some transitional behaviours used in getting to sleep can cause physical damage (pulling out patches of hair, sucking, chewing or biting, causing calloused, reddened or bleeding skin or in extreme cases permanent scarring and tissue damage).

One girl I worked with some years ago at the time she was referred chewed her skin so badly at night that she had exposed tendons on the backs of her hands. Her parents dreaded the bloodstained pillows that greeted them each morning. Her problem responded quickly and effectively using an endorphin-blocking medication coupled with a behavioural programme to redirect her into less distressing activities.

Some transition behaviours can disturb others. I remember one boy referred at age 6 who could only fall asleep rubbing and pulling at his mother's ear, something she had allowed him to do from infancy but found extremely uncomfortable and distracting. This pattern responded well to the introduction of an alternative calming activity and a graded approach to sleeping in his own bed.

Typically these sorts of patterns respond to behavioural interventions – substituting an alternative object or activity and use of a simple reward scheme. This is often easiest to set up with support from a child clinical psychologist or a nurse behavioural therapist.

One study (Miano et al. 2007) compared the use of transitional objects in getting to sleep in a group of ASD children and in age and sex-matched controls (all were aged 3.7–19 years). The authors found no difference between the groups in their use of transitional objects (26% of the ASD group and 18% of controls used transitional objects).

Other factors that can affect sleep

A variety of other factors affect infant sleep. Maternal smoking, for example, has been shown to impair infant arousal (Richardson, Walker and Horne 2009). Maternal alcohol ingestion prior to infant breastfeeding, even at low levels, markedly reduces infant activity during sleep, with compensatory increases in motor activity during subsequent sleep (Mennella and Garcia-Gomez 2001).

Sleep problems in parents and their children are often linked in both normally developing and autistic children. One study (Lopez-Wagner *et al.* 2008) compared parents of autistic and typically developing children using scales to assess both their and their children's sleep. Both groups showed an association between the measures, with a higher rate of difficulties in both parents and children in the autistic group. In the child with autism, any given level of sleep disturbance was associated with greater parental sleep disturbance. This study suggests first, that it could be inherited – an issue that warrants more detailed study, and second, of more immediate practical relevance, help is likely to be of greatest benefit when parent and child problems are addressed in parallel.

HOW MUCH SLEEP IS NORMAL?

A 'typical' night's sleep varies by several hours even in the general population. The length of sleep varies in a variety of ways:

- *By country of residence:* The average person in France sleeps, or at least reports sleeping an hour longer than the average person in Korea and half an hour longer than the average person in the UK.

- *By geographical location (our physical latitude and longitude):* Broadly speaking, problems seem to be greater the further from the equator.

- *By climate:* Differences are reported between populations from the same ethnic background depending on whether they are living in temperate, subtropical or tropical regions and also between different ethnic groups living in the same areas.

Do we need to sleep at all?

The world record for staying awake without artificial stimulants is currently held by Randy Gardner, an American who in 1964 set the record at 264 hours (11 days). This is an exceptional time without sleep, and was presumably exceptional for Randy himself. It is not the upper limit of 'normal' but the upper limit of what has so far been possible.

Some people do seem regularly to require much less or much more sleep than others. It has been recognised for many years that some individuals take very little sleep but without any of the difficulties that would normally be seen if the same sleep pattern was imposed on others: this has been described as 'healthy insomnia'.

Sleep seems to be an essential component of the human day, but there are wide individual variations in the amount that we require. In adults, it has been shown that prolonged sleep loss or restriction impairs the formation of new nerve cells in the hippocampus and interferes with memory (Ferrara *et al.* 2012). This structure is crucial to the formation of new memories. Sleep loss also increases the circulating levels of C-reactive protein, which in turn increases your risk of problems with your heart and circulation.

One rare genetic difference (in a gene called DEC2) has been found in association with shortened sleep but is an unlikely cause of insomnia.

What is a normal sleep pattern for a child?

Our sleep patterns change as we age, as does brain electrical activity, which can also be different in neurodevelopmental disorders like ASD.

There is such a wide variation in what is 'normal' that you might think a child's sleep pattern unusual when it is within the normal range. Knowing what is typical sleep can be important.

As children get older they sleep less. Figure C4 shows the percentages of children at 8, 10 and 12 years of age sleeping for different amounts of time each night. Although the graphs overlap, at 8 years a typical night's sleep is 9–9.5 hours, by 10 it is 8 to 8.5 hours, and by 12 it is down to between 7.5 and 8 hours.

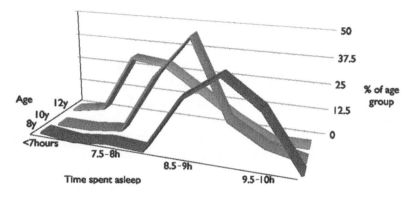

Figure C4: The normal range of sleep in childhood
Source: adapted from Sadeh, Raviv and Gruber 2000

This is based on comparing groups of different ages, however, not on following up the same children. It is easier and quicker to look at large numbers of different children of different ages collected at the same time, but this could mask variation in individuals.

Following the same children over time provides a clearer view of things like stability of individuals' sleep patterns. The average may show gradual changes while individual sleep patterns could change suddenly.

One research group has collected information on sleep patterns and physical growth in a large group of children for over two decades. They have collected regular detailed information on children from the first two years through to 16 (Iglowstein *et al.* 2003).

The amount of sleep gradually reduces with age. At all ages, the normal range is wide – anything between 6 and 12 hours of night-time sleep at 1 year, dropping to between 6.75 and 8.6 hours by 16 years.

One of the most important findings is the wide variation in the amount of sleep seen in normal infants and young children – from less than 6 to more than 14 hours in normal 1-month-olds; this narrows steadily until by 16 years most adolescents are sleeping between 6.75 and 8.5 hours a night.

Girls sleep for longer and make less physical movement while asleep (e.g.: Sadeh *et al.* 2000). This is important to bear in mind when trying to compare studies of children with autism (typically with around 80% boys) against studies of other children (which will usually be 50/50 boys and girls).

It is important not to leap to the assumption that you should be aiming to help your child to achieve some expected typical sleep pattern, especially if this is not typical of your family. A number of sleep issues, like insomnia and familial advanced sleep phase syndrome, are genetic, heritable and result in different sleep patterns to those seen in the general population.

What is a typical night's sleep?

Through the first year of life, night-waking is frequent, and more often than not, the infant requires support to get back to sleep. Without treatment, frequent night-waking is a reasonably stable problem over time that creates increasing strains on families.

The 2004 Sleep in America Poll (Mindell *et al.* 2009) found late bedtime and parental presence in the room while falling asleep were strongly associated with poor child sleep. Neither is necessarily a direct cause – correlation does not prove causation. Parents might stay with a child who is having difficulty falling asleep, and might allow them to stay up later if they don't seem tired or are unlikely to go to sleep when put to bed. It is also possible that the parent's behaviour may be contributing to or even causing the presenting problem.

The later a child goes to bed, the longer they take between going to bed and going to sleep, and the less time they sleep for. When a parent is in the same bedroom, this is associated with more frequent night-waking. In children over 3 years of age, a poor bedtime routine and a television in the bedroom are both associated with shorter sleep. From age 5, consumption of caffeinated soft drinks is also linked.

Part D

REASONS FOR SLEEP PROBLEMS

SLEEP AND MUM'S MOOD

Depression and anxiety are both common issues in parents of people with ASD. These can make consistent parenting more difficult.

Parental mood is a significant predictor of subsequent infant and toddler sleep patterns (O'Connor *et al.* 2007). Higher levels of parental anxiety and depression predict more disturbed child sleep. Developmental difficulties are also more common with low mood in both mother (see: Murray and Cooper 1997) and father (Davé *et al.* 2009).

Infant sleep disturbance can be predicted from levels of maternal distress even before conception (Baird *et al.* 2009). This may reflect the continuing presence of antenatal stress factor/s. There is also mounting evidence for an association between antenatal stressors and the subsequent development of autism (Kinney *et al.* 2008a, 2008b).

Little attention has been paid to the link between parental sleep patterns and child sleep disorders. A study of 2–12-year-old children with sleep difficulties found the complexity of the child's presenting difficulties was greater when parents had excessive daytime sleepiness, with a stronger association to maternal than paternal presentation (Boergers *et al.* 2007). This could merely be that having a child who sleeps poorly stresses mothers out more, but could also indicate a genetic/biological factor that underlies both.

THE BIOLOGY OF SLEEP

A complex biological system underpins our sleep–wake cycles with a specific neuroanatomy, neurochemistry and electrophysiology (see: Rosenwasser 2009). Much of this process is light dependent and ambient light is important in many other aspects of health and disease (Schmoll *et al.* 2010). Other non-light-dependent factors are involved but play minor roles in sleep (Klerman *et al.* 1998).

Differences in melatonin – the chemical that triggers tiredness

Melatonin is a chemical released by the pineal gland, a cone-shaped structure deep in the midbrain. It is sensitive to differences in nocturnal light levels (Zeitzer *et al.* 2000), which explains why simple changes like the use of blackout curtains or phasing out use of a night-light can be effective.

Melatonin supplements mimic the metabolic effects of its natural release (e.g. Braam *et al.* 2009). They can have beneficial effects in circadian rhythm sleep disorders in children with multiple disabilities (Jan and Freeman 2004), when endogenous levels are insufficient to provide a normal sleep trigger. In adults with developmental disabilities lower pre-treatment serum levels of endogenous melatonin predict a positive response (Laasko *et al.* 2007).

A review of melatonin supplements in intellectual disability and sleep disorders (Sajith and Clarke 2007) identified six small studies. Five reported positive results, two with specific clinical groups: Rett syndrome (McArthur and Budden 1998) and tuberous sclerosis (O'Callaghan *et al.* 1999). One study in six children with moderate learning disability failed to report benefit (Camfield *et al.* 1996).

Some people have significantly slower melatonin metabolism than most. Here there is good initial response that tails off rapidly after a few weeks (Braam *et al.* 2010). So far this has only been reported in people with a learning disability, but it has as yet been little studied and may occur more widely. A positive response to supplementation may be re-established through a brief period off supplements, and restarting on a substantially decreased dose.

Melatonin is interesting for several reasons:

- It is a 'chronobiotic' – circulating levels in the bloodstream vary through the day.

- Melatonin is produced from the metabolism of tryptophan (an essential dietary amino acid), by a well-recognised genetic pathway that has been identified as mutated in a number of ASD cases.

- Tryptophan is essential for the production of serotonin, a neurotransmitter also implicated in some cases of ASD, and for which a number of specific genetic factors, linked to ASD, have also been identified (Anderson *et al.* 2009).

- Abnormalities of one melatonin receptor gene, MTNR1B, are overrepresented in the ASD population, suggesting a link between abnormal melatonin binding, ASD and certain types of sleep disorder. MTNR1B is also involved in regulating blood glucose and carrying a mutation increases the risk of type-2 diabetes by around 20%.

- Several studies have identified abnormalities in melatonin production and metabolism in people with ASD (e.g.: Leu *et al.* 2010; Melke *et al.* 2008).

- In some people with ASD, abnormal melatonin synthesis has been shown to be related to reduced activity of the enzyme acetylserotonin methyltransferase (ASMT) (Melke *et al.* 2008). ASMT converts N-acetylserotonin to melatonin the final stage in this biological pathway.

Note: In the USA, melatonin is available as an over-the-counter supplement. In Canada, it is not commonly available. In the UK, it is currently classified as a prescription-only medication – it is classified as 'medicinal by use' as a sleeping aid.

Visual impairments and their link to poor sleep

Retinal damage or dysfunction affects the ability of the brain to modulate melatonin release, as the level of ambient light falling on the retina controls pineal release.

Sleep disturbance is common in individuals who are functionally blind. In the blind, the rate of sleep problems is highest in those with no light perception, or in conditions where the eyes fail to develop (anopthamia: Tabandeh *et al.* 1998).

Impaired vision has often been reported in association with ASD (see, e.g.: Hobson and Bishop 2003). In one large survey, autistic disorder was diagnosed in 30 (approximately 11.7%) of 257 visually impaired 7–18-year-olds (Mukaddes *et al.* 2007).

These findings support the importance of melatonin in the pathogenesis of some cases of ASD. They also give a better understanding of the rationale for the use of melatonin supplementation and an understanding of the neurobiology. The pathways involved in metabolism of serotonin are an important component of the link from diet to behaviour, ASD and sleep issues.

Oxytocin

Oxytocin (a small nine amino acid peptide molecule) has been linked to sleep. It is made by various neurosecretory cells in the hypothalamus and released into the bloodstream from the pituitary gland directly below part of the hypothalamus called the suprachiasmatic nucleus (SCN). The SCN is a key structure involved in governing sleep, and has been called the brain's 'master circadian clock' (Zee and Manthena 2007).

The circadian rhythms of the SCN are affected by a wide range of inputs such as glutamate, pituitary adenylate cyclase activating peptide (PACAP), gamma-aminobutyric acid (GABA), melatonin and neuropeptide Y (see: Reghunandanan and Reghunandanan 2006).

There is much active interest in the role oxytocin plays in EEG mu/ alpha beta rhythms and mirror neuron function (Perry *et al.* 2010). As mu rhythm appears to be important from the earliest stages of social cognition it may be important in the early development of ASD (see: Marshall and Meltzoff 2011).

To date there has been relatively little investigation of the role of oxytocin in sleep, but there is increasing research on its use in ASD. This includes research on a synthetic analogue of oxytocin known as carbetocin, which can be used as a nasal spray. Carbetocin, has recently completed US phase 1 trials as a treatment for the core social impairments in ASD.

Yawning

Some sleep-related behaviours are affected by social context and differ in ASD. Yawning, for example, is 'infectious' – when one person yawns others are more likely to do so (see, e.g.: Provine 1989). This social aspect of yawning is impaired in various conditions including autism (Thompson 2010).

Infectious yawning is a developmental function. In normally developing children it can only be reliably elicited by modelling from around age 5 and by reading or listening to stories about yawning from around 6 (Anderson and Meno 2003).

Yawning can be induced in other animals by observing human yawns. This has been shown in dogs (Joly-Mascheroni, Senju and Shepherd 2008), and can also be seen in other species.

A Japanese study looked at yawning in children watching video of other people yawning or control videos in which no yawning occurred (Senju *et al.* 2007). These were all around 11 years old, 24 with ASD and 25 slightly more cognitively able controls. In the controls, yawning increased when they had watched yawning, in ASD, yawning did not vary by what they saw.

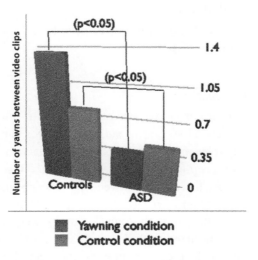

Figure D1: Yawning in autistic children
Source: adapted from Senju et al. 2007

Contagious yawning correlates with empathy and performance on theory of mind tasks – those most likely to yawn when they see someone else yawn also tend to show the strongest empathy and the best abilities to recognise the thoughts, feelings and emotions of others (Platek *et al.* 2003).

The probable biological basis to this system links the visual and limbic system. The structural and functional connectivities involved, between the retinal and hypothalamic systems, are extensive (see: Trachtman 2010).

There is an extensive literature on the associations between sleep and emotion (see: Baglioni *et al.* 2010). Sleep disturbance at age 2 years predicts depressive symptomology at age 10, and could be a useful screening measure for preventative interventions (Gregory *et al.* 2009).

A range of ASD conditions have been shown to have widespread hypothalamic involvement. The ASD conditions so far documented include Biedl-Bardet syndrome, Klinefelter's syndrome, Noonan's syndrome, Prader-Willi syndrome, Rett syndrome, Smith-Magenis syndrome and Tourette's syndrome (see: Aitken 2010a, 2010b).

Diet, sleep and ASD

A number of specific dietary differences have been reported that are potentially relevant to sleep problems.

Low levels of iron intake

Low serum ferritin levels (a measure of iron levels in the blood) have been reported in several studies in autism (see: Dosman *et al.* 2006). This is potentially relevant in sleep problems because one of its effects is disruption to the sleep–wake cycle (see: Lozoff and Georgieff 2006).

There is support for a link between poor sleep and low serum ferritin in ASD (Dosman *et al.* 2007). An open-label study of eight weeks of supplementation with 6mg/kg body weight was carried out. Assessments conducted included pre- and post-treatment blood ferritin, a measure of sleep disturbance and diet recording (Bruni *et al.* 1996). It appears that 69% of the preschoolers and 35% of the school-age children had low dietary iron intake at baseline, and 77% had restless sleep. Both ferritin levels and sleep improved significantly with iron supplementation but there was no significant association between changes on the two measures.

Low levels of dietary tryptophan

Tryptophan is one of nine essential amino acids needed for metabolic processes and that must be taken from your diet.

Tryptophan is converted into 5-HTP by the enzyme tryptophan hydroxylase. Defects in the tryptophan hydroxylase gene, TPH2, have been found in autism (Coon *et al.* 2005). It is rare (Ramoz *et al.* 2006).

This first step in the melatonin pathway needs a co-factor called tetrahydrobiopterin (THBP4). Beneficial effects in autism have been reported in a number of studies, beginning with early Japanese research in the late 1980s, and there has been increasing recent interest (Schnetz-Boutaud *et al.* 2009).

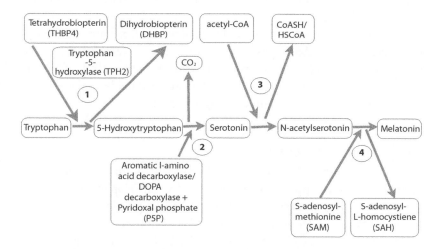

Figure D2: Tryptophan pathway differences in ASD linked to melatonin metabolism and sleep
Key references: 1) Coon et al. *(2005); Schnetz-Boutaud* et al. *(2009); 2) Burlina* et al. *(2001); 3) Weiss* et al. *(2006); 4) Chaste* et al. *(2010); Jonsson* et al. *(2010)*

5-HTP is converted into serotonin by the AADC gene with vitamin B6 as a co-factor. To date only a single case has been reported in which an AADC defect has been linked to ASD (Burlina *et al.* 2001), however relatively few cases of AADC deficiency have been reported and they are usually complex. There is a large literature on the use of B6 supplementation (particularly in the active form, P-5-P), in certain types of refractory seizure activity (see: Baxter 2001) and in ASD.

Serotonin is converted to N-acetylserotonin by an enzyme produced by the gene ITGB3 (Weiss *et al.* 2006). Gene differences have been linked to ASD, and can interact with another gene, SLC6A4 (Coutinho *et al.* 2007), differences which can also elevate serotonin (Coutinho *et al.* 2004).

In the final stage of the pathway, N-acetylserotonin is converted to melatonin using the enzyme acetylserotonin methyltransferase, and the gene controlling its production is abnormal in some ASD families (Melke *et al.* 2008).

Melatonin binds with specific membrane surface receptors, and mutations to several genes coding for these – MTNR1A, MTNR1B, and GPR50 have been associated with ASD (Chaste *et al.* 2010; Jonsson *et al.* 2010).

All of the above steps are under genetic control with differences reported in some ASD cases. Sleep problems may arise from low dietary intake of tryptophan, from problems in the metabolic pathway through which tryptophan is converted into available melatonin, or from differences in melatonin binding receptors.

Excess levels of taurine intake

Taurine is a conditionally essential amino acid that is made from cysteine. Taurine supplements lower blood sugar (Kaplan *et al.* 2004).

Excess taurine ingestion has been linked to problems in two case reports. In one, a 36-year-old man had a manic episode that began after taking taurine, caffeine and inositol which induced an episode of manic behaviour and insomnia (Machado-Vieira, Viale and Kapczinski 2001). In the second, a 27-year-old bodybuilder developed a toxic encephalopathy while taking various supplements including taurine, protein supplements and illegal hormones (Obermann *et al.* 2006).

Taurine is frequently added to energy drinks with increasing concern over emerging links between energy drink consumption and problem behaviour in adolescents (Miller 2008).

Most of the information on problems with taurine use concern its use in combination. Although it is difficult to be clear about specific effects from taurine, as it is likely to be taken in a combination, caution should be exercised not to exceed RDA levels.

Physical factors that can affect sleep

Blood pressure

A group of 238 normal adolescents, without any significant sleep or medical issues, had a variety of recordings: actigraphy, two overnight EEG records and multiple blood pressure measurements to examine associations between demographic factors, blood pressure and sleep quality. Poor sleep was associated with 'pre-hypertensive' blood pressure elevation. Their findings could not be accounted for on the basis of other factors (Javaheri et al. 2008).

With chronic insomnia there is often elevated night-time systolic blood pressure with a smaller daytime to night-time changes. Elevated night-time pressure is correlated with a significant increase in higher frequency EEG activity during non-REM sleep.

Elevated night-time blood pressure may result in poor sleep independently of other factors. Hypertension should be checked in all cases and treated as required if found.

Ear infections and snoring

Ear infections have been suspected as a possible cause of sleep disorders in ASD for some years (Herr 2003).

In a large Kentucky survey (Gozal et al. 2008), recurrent ear infections were almost twice as common in snorers than you would expect if there were no association between the two. The need for tympanostomy (insertion of grommets into the ear to keep the ear canal open) was also increased in the children who snored, suggesting that when snoring and a history of ear infection were both present the ear problems were more severe.

The metabolic syndrome

The 'metabolic syndrome' is the name given to a constellation of clinical features and lifestyle risk factors that increase the risk of diabetes and cardiovascular problems (see, e.g.: Grundy et al. 2004). Currently a variety of overlapping diagnostic criteria are in use. These typically include dyslipidaemia, central obesity, elevated blood pressure and abnormal glucose metabolism.

Sleep apnoea is a recognised secondary problem in paediatric metabolic syndrome (see: Halpern et al. 2010). The co-occurrence of sleep-disordered breathing in adolescents with metabolic syndrome has been reported. In one screening study (Redline *et al.* 2007), 25% of those meeting criteria for metabolic syndrome also had sleep-disordered breathing. This is roughly 6.5 times the expected rate if there were no association.

A significant association has been found in adult community samples between sleep problems and metabolic syndrome (Nieto, Peppard and Young 2009). This is unsurprising as many of the factors reported as part of the metabolic syndrome are also reported with sleep-disordered breathing.

Hypertension, diabetes and insulin resistance, abdominal obesity, and dyslipidaemia are all more common in people with sleep-disordered breathing.

Acid reflux

From adult research, gastrointestinal (GI) problems in general are commonly associated with sleep difficulties. In one series of chronic insomnia patients, 33.6% had GI issues compared to 9.2% of matched controls, and 55.4% of GI patients complained of sleep problems compared to 20.2% of matched controls (Taylor *et al.* 2007).

The GI tract is almost entirely alkaline with the exception of the stomach. The lining of the stomach produces hydrochloric acid and digestive enzymes that are irritating to other tissues in the GI tract.

Gastroesophageal reflux disease, typically called 'GERD', is a condition where acid from the stomach can come up into the throat when someone lies down or takes vigorous exercise. It results from a poorly functioning sphincter at the lower end of the oesophagus (where the upper GI tract joins the top of the stomach). This results in discomfort and physical irritation as the stomach acid irritates and inflames the lining of the oesophagus.

A number of studies have indicated a link between GERD and sleep problems (see: Jung, Choung and Talley 2010). The current view is that the two conditions interact. Difficulties in clearing stomach acid through saliva, swallowing and gastric motility together with adopting a prone position during sleep may aggravate GERD and worsen any problems. These issues are experienced more in the early stages of sleep as reflux reduces during deeper sleep.

The US Sleep Heart Health Study (Fass *et al.* 2005) reported on associations between a large number of variables. They found that sleeping poorly, having an elevated body mass index (BMI) (of 25 or over), insomnia, obstructive sleep apnoea, daytime sleepiness and greater carbonated drink consumption predicted heartburn during sleep. This was strongly associated with GERD.

One study in 25 older adults with GERD (mean age 42.8) examined the effects of a specific medication, rabeprazole (which reduces acid production by the stomach) (Orr *et al.* 2009). An eight-week course of treatment produced significant improvement in upper airway function and in sleep quality on objective measurement and on patient ratings. Rabeprazole is not currently approved in the USA or the UK for use under 18 years of age.

A possible link between ASD and GERD is suggested by a clinical case series from Baltimore (Horvath *et al.* 1999). This report was on upper endoscopy (examining the throat as far as the entrance to the stomach with a fibre-optic device). They studied 36 children with autism and GI issues. GERD was reported as a common finding in ASD, associated with a high rate of sleep disorders. That a condition that causes pain and discomfort on lying down tends to co-occur with sleeping problems should not come as any surprise.

Inflammatory biomarkers and related immune issues

Various immune factors affect sleep (see: Imeri and Opp 2009; Krueger 2008). Some are increased when you have an infection and may underlie the change in sleep patterns seen at such times.

Immune differences are found in ASD (see, e.g.: Ashwood *et al.* 2011). Measurement is complex because immune markers vary with age (see: Sack *et al.* 1998) and sex (Sadeghi *et al.* 2005). One recent study of children with ASD found daytime elevation of plasma cytokine levels (Ashwood *et al.* 2011). No published study has so far correlated immune factors that are reportedly different in ASD, such as TNF-a and IL-6, with sleep disturbance.

We know that in the lab sleep deprivation alters immune markers like TNF-a receptor 1 and interleukin-6; c-reactive protein; and interleukin-17. Changes in interleukin-6 caused by sleep restriction are strongly associated with increased pain perception. The increase in c-reactive protein, which is coupled with increased heart rate can be brought on by sleep restriction. The effects last well after sleep has recovered and increase cardiopulmonary risk. These suggest some of these immune differences may be reactive rather than constitutional, could be secondary to persistent sleep difficulties and that they might improve if sleep difficulties were corrected.

The processes are complex with increases in both pro- and anti-inflammatory markers. Increases in c-reactive protein and interleukin-6 are associated with increased sleep while increases in TNF-a are associated with reduced sleep.

Many other things can influence inflammatory markers (see: O'Connor *et al.* 2009 for discussion), and strong conclusions are premature. Obstructive sleep apnoea (OSA), for example, is associated with an increase in the levels of pro-inflammatory markers, but as is also strongly associated with obesity, asthma control and cardiopulmonary difficulties, making it difficult to establish which affects which.

Other factors that can influence sleep

Skin issues

Increased melatonin intake from breastfeeding can improve allergic dermatitis (Kimata 2001, 2004). There is no similar effect from bottle-feeds, which do not typically contain melatonin.

Psoriasis and other dermatological conditions that increase itchiness and scratching are more common in those with sleeping difficulties (see: Jafferany 2007). These problems can sometimes arise as a consequence of medications given to help with comorbid conditions such as ADHD, seizures or mood swings.

Surprisingly little good research has been carried out on the possible links between skin problems and sleep (see: Thorburn and Riha 2010).

Epilepsy

Sleep problems are common in people with epilepsy (see, e.g.: Manni and Terzaghi 2010; Matos *et al.* 2010) and epilepsy is often seen in people with ASD.

The association between epilepsy and sleep issues is thought to result from a similarity in the 'oscillatory patterns' involved, with epileptic discharges developing from sleep-related patterns (Beenhakker and Huguenard 2009).

Some children who have been diagnosed with night terrors have instead been found to have night-time seizures (see, e.g.: Lombroso 2000).

One large study (Byars *et al.* 2008) examined the interrelationships between neuropsychological functioning and sleep problems in children with recent seizures. Settling difficulties, daytime sleepiness and parasomnias were significantly more common in comparison both to sibling controls and to typical rates. Difficulties shown on neuropsychological testing were strongly associated with sleep problems.

Fluctuations through the sleep–wake cycle are involved in a range of changes to brain functioning including synaptic plasticity. On this basis, fluctuation in seizure threshold may vary depending on factors like sleep state and sleep deprivation (Romcy-Pereira, Leite and Garcia-Cairasco 2009).

SLEEP DEPRIVATION AND BRAIN GROWTH

The hippocampus is a brain structure easily damaged by low oxygen levels. It is critical to a range of CNS processes including memory formation and stabilising glucose levels.

In humans even relatively brief periods of sleep restriction can have marked effects on cognitive function. In a study comparing performance of 16 children aged 1 to 14 years, allowed either 5 or 11 hours of time in bed in a sleep laboratory, Randazzo *et al.* (1998) found the children who experienced restricted sleep, although not impaired on simple cognitive tasks or rote learning, were impaired on tests of verbal creativity, mental flexibility and executive functioning.

Sleep problems often begin at times of active brain development (i.e. during processes like neural proliferation, dendritic arborisation, dendritic pruning or apoptosis) and might be expected to affect it. Brain development is most active in early childhood and during early adolescence (Casey, Duhoux and Cohen 2010).

BRAIN INJURIES

Rates of sleep disorder are also higher in people who have experienced CNS trauma (Makley *et al.* 2008; Rao *et al.* 2008). Traumatic injuries, particularly to the head, are more frequent than expected in ASD (McDermott, Zhou and Mann 2008) and are associated with high rates of post-injury anxiety and depression (Whelan-Goodinson *et al.* 2009).

ATTENTION-DEFICIT HYPERACTIVITY DISORDER (ADHD)

(See, for reviews: Owens 2005; Mayes et al. 2009.)

ASD and ADHD are often seen in the same individual and there is a high degree of symptom overlap (see: Ponde, Novaes and Losapio 2010). Stimulant medications are frequently used with such children. The possibility that sleep issues are a side-effect should always be considered, especially if they began after starting medication.

Some sleep problems are more common in ADHD: particularly restless legs syndrome and sleep-disordered breathing (Cortese, Konofal and Yateman, 2006; O'Brien et al. 2003a). In addition, periodic limb movement syndrome and narcolepsy also seem to be overrepresented (see, for discussion: Owens 2005).

Rates of sleep disorders are high in children with ADHD (Gruber, Sadeh and Raviv 2000; Mayes et al. 2009; Walters et al. 2008). This may be an effect of constitutional make-up or a direct consequence of stimulant medication (Berman et al. 2009; Corkum et al. 2008; O'Brien et al. 2003b; Sangal et al. 2006). With few exceptions (see, e.g.: Faraone et al. 2009) sleep disturbance, or the exacerbation of pre-existing sleep difficulties, is reported in children and adolescents being treated with stimulant medication for ADHD symptomology.

Snoring is three times as common in paediatric ADHD as in other psychiatric groups or in the general population, affecting some 33% (O'Brien et al. 2003a). If effectively treated, typically by removal of the tonsils and adenoids, 50% no longer meet ADHD criteria (Chervin et al. 2006). Unfortunately, for a significant subgroup, adenotonsilectomy does not stop the snoring (Liukkonen et al. 2008).

PHYSICAL GROWTH AND SLEEP

Sleeping problems can be more common when the skull or facial muscles develop abnormally. In 'hemifacial microsomia', one side of the face and skull develop more slowly and are significantly smaller than the other (this is seen in various conditions such as Goldenhar's syndrome). This may interfere with breathing and increase the risk of apnoea (Hui 2009).

Differences in throat and mouth development can affect their structure and function and, together with the size of the lungs, the development of the muscles and the level of body fat, increases the chance of developing OSA.

OBESITY

A link between obesity and sleep difficuties is common (Van Cauter and Knutson 2008), and is reported in various adult (Bjorvatn *et al.* 2007; Patel *et al.* 2006) and child (Reilly *et al.* 2005; Seicean *et al.* 2007) studies. The association has not been universally accepted (see, e.g.: Mehra and Redline 2008).

Poor sleep interferes with normal metabolism which in turn affects sleep quality. Poor sleep is linked to obesity, impairing insulin output with a greater incidence and severity of obstructive sleep apnoea and type-2 diabetes (see: Trenell, Marshall and Rogers 2007).

GENETIC CONDITIONS WITH HIGH RATES OF SLEEP PROBLEMS

Sleep problems are more common in a number of genetic syndromes (Table D1). In particular, Prader-Willi syndrome, Angelman syndrome, Down syndrome, Rett syndrome, Smith-Magenis syndrome and, much more rarely, Kleine-Levin syndrome are genetic conditions reported in association with ASD. All frequently present with sleep disorders (see, for review: Aitken 2010a, 2010b).

Table D1: Genetic conditions in ASD associated with sleep problems

Condition	Gene locus/loci	Key references
Prader-Willi syndrome	5q11–q13; 15q12	Bruni, Verrillo, Novelli and Ferri (2010b); Cotton and Richdale (2010)
Kleine-Levin syndrome	6p21.3	Berthier, Santamaria, Encabo, Tolosa (1992)
Angelman syndrome	15q11–q13; Xq28	Pelc, Cheron, Boyd and Dan (2008)
Smith-Magenis syndrome	17p11.2	De Leersnyder, Claustrat, Munnich and Verloes (2006)
Down syndrome	Trisomy 21	Diomedi *et al.* (1999); Cotton and Richdale (2006, 2010)
Rett syndrome	Xq28	Rohdin *et al.* (2007)

'Clock genes'

Our genetic make-up specifies 'invariant features' of our bodies, how they are built and how they function. 'Homeobox'/HOX genes specify the physical layout of our bodies (Holland, Booth and Bruford 2007) and have been 'conserved' over evolution, virtually unchanged in structure and function (see: Garcia-Fernàndez 2005). They specify things like patterning of body parts, their midline symmetry (many structures show symmetry – brains, eyes, nostrils, arms, legs, ribs, kidneys, lungs and genitals, to name a few). A few organ systems – the liver, intestines and heart, for example – do not show this pattern of gross structural symmetry.

Many other aspects of our bodies are genetically specified. Predictable biological rhythms, from resting heart rate and breathing pattern to circadian and ultradian rhythms, have genetic bases. These are less easy to see and have taken longer to identify. From our coordination, how we move in social interaction, to our heartbeats and our sleep patterns we are partly at least controlled by 'clock genes' (see: Bamne *et al.* 2010).

Clock genes modulate brain systems involving synaptic cell adhesion molecules and post-synaptic scaffolding proteins that provide the internal timing of synaptic functions (see: Toro *et al.* 2010), controlling temporal changes in our brains that parallel diurnal changes in the environment.

Abnormalities in some clock genes have been found in sleep disorders (reviewed in Ebisawa 2007). They may also have roles in other conditions such as metabolic syndrome and breast cancer. The hypothalamic-pituitary-adrenal axis is affected by clock genes (Nader, Chrousos and Kino 2010) and may affect appetite and risk of obesity (Yang *et al.* 2009).

Clock gene anomalies may be associated both with difficulties seen in autistic social interactions and with the high rate of reported sleeping problems in ASD (Wimpory, Nicholas and Nash 2002).

Seasonally changing rates of sleep problems are seen in the general population (see, e.g.: Pallesen *et al.* 2001) and in ASD (Hayashi 2001).

Fifteen genes involved in the regulation of circadian rhythm have been identified that frequently show quantitative or qualitative differences in ASD (Hu *et al.* 2009; Nicholas *et al.* 2007) (Table D2).

Table D2: Clock gene differences in ASD

Clock gene	Gene locus	Association with ASD (+/-)	Key reference
Per3	1p36.23	+	Hu *et al.* (2009)
Npas2	2q13	+	Nicholas *et al.* (2007)
BHLHb2/DEC1	3q25.1	?	Hu *et al.* (2009)
Clock	4q21	+	Hu *et al.* (2009)
RORA	15q22.2	+	Nguyen *et al.* (2010)
Per1	17p12	+	Nicholas *et al.* (2007)

Some clock gene differences are linked to specific sleep problems. A Per3 length polymorphism has been reported in association with delayed sleep phase syndrome (Archer *et al.* 2003).

CONCLUSION

Some sleep problems are simple, some are complex, some are common to ASD while others are rare. A wide range of approaches is available, some of which can be carried out without any assistance while others will require clinical help and supervision. As for so much else, one size does not fit all.

Some issues like poor sleep hygiene respond to general interventions that should be easy to implement and help in many cases. This is often not enough. Many of the approaches we have discussed will help only for specific problems. I have stressed throughout the importance of good observation, collecting a baseline, being clear about the problem and finding the correct diagnosis. You will need to keep good records, be clear about what was done and about the results.

Sleep difficulties in ASD is an area with a rapidly growing evidence base. What is best practice today may not be best practice next month. Better information improves and changes practice. This short volume gives an up-to-date summary of best practice at the time of writing, and how to keep track of progress in this area. I hope it will help many people dealing with these often confusing, perplexing and exhausting problems to find answers.

GLOSSARY

I have not included medications or herbal treatments in this glossary as the relevant ones are indexed and covered in the appendices. As there are many uncommon terms used in describing sleep disorders, a basic glossary seemed essential.

> One reason why other people find it hard to understand science, and why scientists are apt to lose their tempers with other people, is that scientists use ordinary words with a special meaning, or invent words of their own which ordinary people do not understand. (Haldane 1927, p.161)

Acetylserotonin methyltransferase (ASMT) The enzyme that catalyses the reaction converting n-acetylserotonin into melatonin.

Actigraphy An automated method of recording movement during sleep, usually through a wrist recorder that registers movement.

Adenosine A nucleic acid found in DNA and RNA. It can also function as a neurotransmitter. It is composed of adenine and d-ribose.

Adenosine triphosphate (ATP) An adenine nucleotide with three phosphate groups that is involved in mitochondrial energy production. In addition it functions as a neurotransmitter and is involved in muscle activity through ATP dependent myosins.

Adrenocorticotropic hormone (ACTH) A hormone secreted by the pituitary gland that affects the production of cortical steroids by the adrenal glands.

Agonist A compound that acts to increase the available levels of another biologically active substance.

Apnoea (Apnea) A brief period when someone stops breathing.

Apoptosis Selective programmed cell death as a means of refining brain function.

Aromatic amino acid (AADC) The lyase enzyme that converts 5-HTP to serotonin (5-hydroxytryptophan carboxylase I-decarboxylase).

Ascending reticular activating system (ARAS) The ARAS is a midbrain system that regulates our state of arousal.

Astrocyte The largest and most prolific glial cells in the nervous system. They have projections in all directions, hence the name, derived from the Greek word *ástron* meaning star.

Atonia Sleep paralysis, a condition where the person is awake and aware but unable to make voluntary movements.

B6 One of the B vitamins, aka pyridoxal. Its active form, pyridoxal phosphate (P-5-P), is involved in many aspects of amino acid metabolism including production of serotonin.

B12 A B-vitamin, a.k.a. cobalamin, it is a cobalt-based compound with a structure not unlike haemoglobin. It is involved in a wide range of bodily processes from DNA synthesis, fatty acid and blood production to brain function.

Bell and pad see: Enuresis alarm

Body mass index (BMI) The BMI is a number (a person's weight divided by the square of their height; this is sometimes called the 'Quetelet index'). It is used as a proxy figure for body fat compared to the general population.

Bruxism Tooth-grinding – habitual involuntary grinding or clenching of the teeth.

CAP A fluctuating pattern seen in the unstable phases of NREM sleep.

CAT scan A computerised axial tomography (or CAT) scan enables information from an X-ray source rotated around an object to be built up, giving a cross-sectional image. This was the first technique that allowed imaging of brain structures in situ.

Cataplexy A sudden loss of muscle tone and voluntary control brought on by a strong emotion such as fear or shock or an unexpected noise or movement.

Catathrenia Sleep-related groaning.

Chronobiotic A substance or process that varies systematically over the 24-hour period.

Chronotype This term is used to classify people according to their daily rhythms – typically into groups who are at their best in the morning or evening.

Circadian Processes that typically follow a 24-hour cycle.

Circadian Rhythm Sleep Disorder A group of conditions that cause disruption to the time pattern of sleep rather than to the production of sleep itself. DSM-5 differentiates between a number of specific types:

- delayed sleep phase type (with a significant delay in sleeping and waking on most nights)
- jet lag type (transient and induced by long-distance air travel across time zones)
- shift work type (insomnia and/or excessive sleepiness in people who work irregular hours that interfere with the person's normal sleep pattern
- free-running type (also called non-entrained type; non-24-hour sleep–wake syndrome and hypernychthemeral syndrome) is a regular daily sleep–wake pattern that is longer than 24 hours in which the person gradually desynchronises and resynchronises with the day–night pattern)
- irregular sleep–wake type (in which there is a variable sleep pattern with sleepiness alternating with insomnia).

Clock genes Genes whose expression varies through the day dependent on other circadian processes.

CNS central nervous system.

Coeliac An allergic reaction to gluten that can be tested for (people with coeliac disease have anti-endomesial and anti-gliadin antibodies).

Coercive family process When family members control each other's behaviours by doing things that neither likes but both engage in as a learned response to the other.

Co-factor A co-factor is an additional compound required for a metabolic process to work effectively.

Conservation A gene is conserved if it is unchanged across a range of species. It is assumed that lack of change is an indication that the gene specifies a process that has broad biological importance and the wider the range (say a gene was the same in all species from amoebae to man), the greater its significance and the earlier it evolved.

Cortisol A steroid hormone produced by the adrenal glands that increases in response to stress, elevating blood sugar levels.

CPAP (continuous positive airway pressure) This is a method of treating obstructive sleep apnoea by wearing a device (typically a face mask connected to a machine) that delivers air at higher pressure to the person while they are sleeping. The increased air pressure keeps the airways open, making breathing easier and typically reducing or eliminating snoring.

Cycling alternating pattern see: CAP.

Dendritic arborisation The growth of dendrites occurring as a network is strengthened through use.

Dendritic pruning The reduction in dendrites resulting from lack of use.

Dream sleep see: REM sleep.

DTI (diffusion tensor) A form of MRI imaging that extracts information on imaging interrelationships across different structures in the nervous system based on fractional anisotropy.

Dyslipidaemia A term for abnormally low or high levels of lipids in the bloodstream. Typically used to mean elevated levels.

Dyssomnias Sleep disorders that make getting to sleep and/or staying asleep more difficult than normal.

EEG A system for recording of electrical (electro-encephalogram) activity from the brain by using pairs of surface electrodes that are attached to the scalp. This enables the different stages of sleep to be monitored and identified and could also identify some types of epileptic activity as they occur.

EMG (electro-myography) Recording of muscular activity using surface electrodes.

Empathy The ability to recognise and relate to the feelings of others.

Enuresis Involuntary urination beyond the age when bladder control is typically achieved.

Enuresis alarm A device that is triggered by voiding (passing urine) resulting in the completion of an electric circuit that in turn is used to trigger a means of rousing the person – typically a buzzer/bell but this can be a vibrating mat radio or other device that could bring the person to a waking state.

Epiphenomenon An association that occurs consistently but which does not have causal or biological significance.

Extinction A means of reducing a learned response to a cue that was previously paired with an undesired situation. In this context, the child who has been used to parent attention for noisy behaviour on being put to bed (the learned response) is ignored until quiet and rewarded once settled (pairing the desired behaviour with the expected outcome).

Ferritin A protein complex found throughout the body that stores and releases iron.

FMRI Functional magnetic resonance imaging is a technique for imaging metabolic activity by using the proxy measure of changes in blood flow.

FRAXTAS Fragile-X associated tremor/ataxia syndrome is a recently recognised late-onset motor condition first reported in the maternal grandfathers of boys with Fragile-X syndrome.

Functional analysis A detailed description and analysis of behaviour that tries to identify the factors maintaining a particular pattern of responses.

GABA (gamma-aminobutyric acid) GABA is an inhibitory neurotransmitter that regulates muscle tone.

GERD A condition in which gastric juices from the stomach (gastroesophageal) are brought up the oesophagus resulting in irritation reflux disease and inflammation of the lining of the throat. GERD is the most common acronym as much of the research on the condition is carried out in the USA, it can also be referred to as gastro-oesophageal reflux disease (GORD) using the spelling more common in the UK; gastric reflux disease; or as acid reflux disease.

Ghrelin A recently identified sleep- and appetite-controlling hormone produced primarily by the stomach with receptors in the pituitary and hypothalamus.

Glia A class of non-neuronal cells that is part of the nervous system.

Gluten A protein derived mainly from wheat, barley, rye and other related grains.

Glycogen A polysaccharide that constitutes the major carbohydrate energy reserve of the body, stored primarily in liver and muscle tissue.

Graduated extinction As for extinction, defined above, except that bedtime tantrums are ignored, with periodic reassurance, gradually extending the periods between re-settling.

Growth hormone A pituitary peptide hormone involved in a range of processes affecting cell growth and differentiation that is secreted primarily during Stage 3 sleep.

Head-banging Self-injurious behaviour typically involving hitting the head against the headboard, the wall or into the pillow.

Hemifacial microsomia A condition in which one side of the face has grown to a lesser extent than the other. Goldenhaar's syndrome is the best-known example.

Hertz A measure of the number of times a pattern repeats or cycles every second; in this context it measures the speed of the electrical activity recorded from the brain by an EEG.

Holmes, Sherlock The fictional detective in the stories of Arthur Conan Doyle (1859–1930), a Scottish doctor and writer, who showcased the problem-solving approach to forensic medicine.

Hypercalcuria Elevated urinary calcium levels.

Hypersomnia Excessive sleepiness, usually during daytime hours.

Hypertension Elevated blood pressure.

Hypnagogic hallucination Vivid dream-like hallucinations that are said to occur as someone is falling asleep.

Hypocretin see: Orexin.

Hypopnoa A transient period of shallow breathing occurring for 10 seconds or more that occurs while asleep.

Hyposomnia Where someone sleeps at night for significantly shorter amounts of time than normal.

Hypothalamic-pituitary-adrenal axis A closely integrated system that is involved in various processes including adaptation to stress, sleep, digestion and immune function.

Hypothalamus A deep midbrain structure, lying below the thalamus that is the main centre for control of the autonomic nervous system.

Insomnia When a person or their caregiver complains about a sleep problem involving difficulty getting to sleep; frequent night-waking with problems getting back to sleep; early morning waking or feeling unrested on waking.

Insulin A large pancreatic hormone that regulates glucose metabolism.

Interneurons Nerve cells whose axon and dendrites lie completely within the central nervous system, often linking afferent and efferent systems.

ITGB3 A gene for the ß3 subunit of the platelet membrane adhesive protein receptor complex that has recently been shown to be involved in control of male serotonin levels.

Jactatio capitis nocturna Head-banging that occurs during sleep.

'K complexes' A high-voltage waveform seen in Stage 2 sleep. Observed to occur more frequently than normal in RLS and less frequently in OSA. Present from 5 months and increasingly common through adolescence.

Ketogenic diet A diet low in refined sugars and carbohydrates that causes the body to increase its conversion of fats for energy – this has the additional consequence of making ketones which are excreted in urine.

Ketone Ketones are a group of compounds in which a carbonyl group is bonded to two others. Acetone is the best known. In the current context, ketones are compounds excreted when triglyceride fats are broken down to provide energy.

Kleine-Levin syndrome A rare genetic condition which is usually first noticed in adolescence. It presents with sudden-onset lengthy periods of sleep, excessive eating, disinhibition, irritability and hypersexual behaviour.

Leptin A hormone involved in regulation of energy metabolism that is mainly synthesised from white adipose tissue with a circadian release pattern.

MAD (mandibular advancement device) A device to hold the lower jaw and the tongue forward in an attempt to make breathing easier and reduce snoring.

Melatonin An endocrine hormone released in a circadian pattern by the pineal gland. It is involved in initiation of sleep.

Metabolic syndrome A pattern of features associated with increased risks of cardiovascular diseases and type-2 diabetes. A number of diagnostic criteria are in use; common features are usually taken as central obesity, dyslipidaemia and raised blood pressure.

MRI (magnetic fields resonance imaging) A method of imaging that uses strong magnetic fields to align atoms in lower molecular weight molecules, aligning the magnetisation using radio frequency. In human imaging this process allows clear imaging of softer tissues that are high in lower weight molecules such as water.

MSLT (multiple sleep latency test) A standardised test, normally involving an overnight sleep study and the following day, four or five daytime scheduled sleep opportunities, usually over a period of around seven hours, during which a number of things are monitored including EEG, muscle activity and eye movements.

Mu rhythm An EEG pattern that fluctuates in the 8–12 Hertz band. The pattern normally disappears when watching someone else's actions.

Myotonic dystrophy A common form of muscular dystrophy, usually developing in adults, but with a milder type of the DM1 form (aka Steinert's dystrophy/disease) which has been reported in association with ASD developing in childhood.

N-acetylserotonin The intermediate molecule produced in making melatonin from serotonin.

Narcolepsy A condition which is characterised by sudden uncontrollable compulsion to sleep at odd times.

Narcolepsy-cataplexy A complex sleep disorder with excessive daytime sleepiness, sudden loss of muscle tone, sleep paralysis. Thought to result from a genetic deficiency in the production of orexin.

Neuropeptide Y A hypothalamic peptide neurotransmitter involved in a range of functions including energy balance, food intake and circadian rhythm.

Nightmares Dreams with frightening, horrible or distressing content that are remembered on waking.

Night terrors/sleep terrors (aka *pavor nocturnus*) Extreme fear and agitation when waking from non-REM sleep that is not associated with dream recall.

Nocturia The need to urinate frequently at night.

Nocturnal enuresis Urinating during sleep – typically presenting as bedwetting.

Nocturnal seizures Epileptic seizures that occur during sleep.

NREM Non-rapid eye movement phases of sleep.

NTI (Nociceptive trigeminal inhibition) splint A device that alters the movement of the lower jaw, redirecting it forwards and twisting. This is an uncomfortable movement that should deter bruxism.

Obesity Excessive accumulation of body fat to a level where it has begun to compromise the person's physical health.

Obstructive sleep apnoea (OSA) A breathing problem that results in snoring during sleep, often associated with obesity.

Obstructive sleep apnoea-hypopnoea syndrome A sleep pattern characterised by periods of apnoea (breathing stopping due to the throat collapsing while asleep) or hypopnoea (restricted breathing) during sleep.

Occlusal splint A moulded cover for the upper or lower teeth that prevents tooth-grinding.

'Off label' use The use of a prescription medication, under consultant supervision, for a purpose for which it has not been licensed or recommended ('off-license').

Orexin A strongly conserved pair of neuropeptide hormones, also called hypocretins. They have been found to play a major role in the control of wakefulness.

Oxytocin A peptide hormone produced by the hypothalamus that is involved in social behaviour.

Parasomnias Sleep disorders in which there are unusual movements, emotions, behaviours, perceptions or reported dreams.

Paroxetine A medication known as a selective serotonin reuptake inhibitor, typically used as an antidepressant.

Periodic limb movements in sleep (PLMS) Rhythmic leg movements during sleep are seen in more than 1 in 20 adults. They are uncommon in children but can be seen in association with sleep apnoea. These are often not noticed until the person has a polysomnography record.

PET Positron emission tomography, the first useful method of *in vivo* functional neuroimaging.

Phasic REM The phasic stages of REM sleep coincide with higher levels of eye movement and dream recall. The arousal threshold is similar to that seen in Stage 3 sleep.

Pineal gland A tiny endocrine structure situated between the thalamic nuclei at the base of the brain which releases melatonin in a circadian pattern affected by retinal input on ambient light levels.

Pituitary adenylate A hormone with actions on the nervous and gastrointestinal systems.

Plasma The yellowish liquid that is the fluid component of human blood and carries red blood cells.

Polysomnography An assessment of various functions including EEG, eye movements, heart and respiratory rate, pulse oximetry and skeletal muscle activity carried out during sleep.

Ponderal index A measure of body proportions calculated as the relationship between mass and length.

Positive reinforcement Systematic reward that increases the probability of recurrence of behaviour that preceded it.

Prazosin One of a class of medications known as an 'alpha-blocker', prazosin is an anxiolytic – it relaxes the walls of blood vessels and lowers blood pressure.

Prolactin A circadian peptide hormone released by the pituitary gland with levels correlated with amount of REM sleep. Typically associated with its role in stimulating breast milk production after birth.

Pyridoxal phosphate (P5P) The biologically active form of vitamin B6.

RCT (randomised controlled trial) A type of research where matched subjects are allocated at random to different groups to examine the effects of specific differences in treatment on outcome.

REM sleep Rapid eye movement/paradoxical sleep is a specific sleep stage during which most dreams appear to be recalled. Characterised by intense waking-like cortical activation with a lack of muscular movement apart from the eyes.

Restless legs syndrome (RLS) A condition in which lying still results in an uncomfortable sensation in the legs. It is present while awake but commonly seen as part of a sleep problem. First described by the Swedish neurologist Karl Ekbom in 1945.

S-adenosyl-l-homocysteine (SAH) SAH is produced from SAM in the production of melatonin.

S-adenosyl methionine (SAM) A compound, primarily active in liver, with a variety of metabolic functions, one of which is to catalyse the conversion of N-acetylserotonin to melatonin.

Scaffolding proteins Proteins involved in co-factor binding during gene transcription.

SCFAs (short-chain acids) Fatty acids with aliphatic tails of less than six carbons. They are directly absorbed through the hepatic portal vein into the liver and are produced by digestion of dietary fibre.

Scheduled awakening An approach in which the child is gently and deliberately wakened and re-settled.

SDB (sleep-disordered breathing) A range of changes in breathing pattern which can be associated with disorders such as snoring and OSA.

Sensori-motor rhythm An oscillating EEG pattern typically of 12–14 Hertz (SMR) that can be recorded during Stage 2 sleep.

Serotonin A key neurotransmitter, derived from tryptophan, and a precursor of melatonin. Important in regulation of gastrointestinal motility, and important in mood, appetite, muscle contraction and sleep.

Serum Blood plasma with the coagulants removed.

Setting events Aspects of the individual or the environment that constrain the behaviours that can occur around the sleep problem.

Sleep A recurrent pattern in the behaviour of all higher species so far studied. In humans, it is a daily pattern that lasts several hours during which we are inactive and largely unresponsive to external events. It is accompanied by a characteristic pattern of brain activity and body chemistry not seen at other times.

Sleep efficiency This is a measure of how well someone is sleeping. It is usually estimated as: Number of minutes asleep $\times$ 100 $\div$ Number of minutes in bed with the light out.

Sleep hygiene Control of the behaviour and factors that occur in the time leading up to sleep that influence its onset, length and quality.

Sleep spindles Bursts of EEG activity generated by the thalamus during Stage 2 sleep that correspond to muscle twitches.

Sleepwalking (somnambulism) Movements during deep sleep that can include walking and other activities that would normally be performed while fully awake.

Snoring Noises made by vibration of the soft palate caused by breathing during sleep, more commonly associated with obesity.

SNRI (serotonin-norepinephrine inhibitor) A class of medications that increase the circulating levels of the neurotransmitters serotonin and reuptake norepinephrine. Most frequently used in clinical practice as antidepressants.

Social Stories™ Picture sequences used, together with simple verbal descriptions, to help a child with ASD to cope with a situation, develop a skill or grasp a concept. Developed by the US clinician Carol Gray.

Somnambulism see: Sleepwalking.

Somniloquy Talking during sleep.

SPECT (Single-Photon Emission Computerised Tomography) SPECT is an imaging technique that relies on detection of an injected radionucleotide (typically with a tagged form of oxygen). It is similar to PET scanning. SPECT provides lower resolution information but the approach is easier to develop as it uses isotopes 99mTc-HMPAO that are slower to degrade and do not require access to a local cyclotron and isotope processing facility.

SSRI (selective serotonin reuptake inhibitor) A class of medications that increase the circulating levels of the serotonin by reducing reabsorption of serotonin from the post-synaptic cleft after a serotonergic nerve cell has fired. Frequently used in clinical practice as antidepressants.

Stridor A high-pitched wheezing sound made when someone is breathing in.

Superior temporal gyrus The upper surface of the temporal lobe of the brain, containing the primary auditory cortex. It contains Wernicke's area, a key area that enables us to process the spoken language of others.

Suprachiasmatic nucleus A small area of the brain directly above the optic chiasm (where the nerve tracts from the retinas join). It is a key structure in the neural and neurochemical control of circadian rhythms.

Systolic blood pressure The maximum blood pressure during a heartbeat.

Taurine A sulphur-containing amino acid that is derived from cysteine. It is found in the digestive system in bile. The name comes from the Greek word for bull because it was first identified in an extract from ox bile.

Testosterone An androgen steroid hormone primarily secreted by the testes in males and ovaries in females. It shows a strong circadian pattern in men.

THBP4 (tetrahydro-biopterin) An important co-factor in the degradation of phenylalanine and the production of a range of neurotransmitters.

Thyroid stimulating hormone A circadian pituitary peptide hormone involved in the control of thyroid function.

Tonic REM This term is used to classify the periods of REM sleep that occur between phasic bursts of rapid eye movements. The arousal threshold during tonic REM is similar to that during Stage 2 sleep.

Tooth-grinding see: Bruxism.

Transitional objects Physical objects (typically blankets, soothers and soft toys) used by infants to help them to cope, typically at times when primary caregiver contact is not possible.

Tryptophan An essential amino acid critical for the production of serotonin and melatonin.

Tryptophan hydroxylase An enzyme which catalyses the reaction by which THBP4 and oxygen converts tryptophan to 5HTP with iron as a co-factor.

Tympanostomy Surgical insertion of a grommet (a small tube) into the ear canal to hold it open and improve hearing.

Tyrosine hydroxylase An enzyme that limits the production of the neurotransmitter dopamine.

Ultradian Processes that typically follow a cycle repeating within a day.

UP3/UPPP (uvulopalatopharyngoplasty) A complex surgical procedure to widen the back of the throat in an effort to make breathing easier. It is used with OSA. Only the more complex 'Stanford protocol' has been reported to have a high rate of success.

Vasopressin A peptide hormone, produced in the paraventricular and supraoptic nuclei in the pituitary gland. It is similar in structure to oxytocin. Vasopressin controls blood pressure and kidney function.

Videosomnography Video-recording of the person during sleep to monitor REM and body movement.

Videotelemetry A method that combines video-recording of behaviour with EEG recording of brain activity (an explanatory leaflet can be downloaded from www. brainandspine.org.uk).

Zebrafish The zebrafish, *Danio rerio*, is a common subject for genetic research. Its genome has been fully sequenced, a number of well-studied genetic mutants are available for study and it has a well-documented range of predictable behaviours.

REFERENCES

Adams, J.B. and Holloway, C. (2004) 'Pilot study of a moderate dose multivitamin/ mineral supplement for children with autistic spectrum disorder.' *Journal of Alternative and Complementary Medicine, 10*(6): 1033–1039.

Advisory Committee on Childhood Lead Poisoning Prevention (ACCLPP) (2000) 'Recommendations for blood lead screening of young children enrolled in Medicaid: Targeting a group at high risk.' *CDC MMWR, 49*(RR-14): 1–14.

Ailouni, K.M., Ahmad, A.T., El-Zaheri, M.M., Ammari, F.L. *et al.* (2005) 'Sleepwalking associated with hyperthyroidism.' *Endocrine Practice, 11*(4): 5–10.

Ainsworth, M.D.S., Blehar, M.C., Waters, E., and Wall, S. (1978) *Patterns of Attachment: A Psychological Study of the Strange Situation.* Hillsdale, NJ: Lawrence Erlbaum.

Aitken, K.J. (2008) *Dietary Interventions in Autism Spectrum Disorders: Why They Work When They Do, Why They Don't When They Don't.* London: Jessica Kingsley Publishers.

Aitken, K.J. (2010a) *An A–Z of the Genetic Factors in Autism: A Handbook for Parents and Carers.* London: Jessica Kingsley Publishers.

Aitken, K.J. (2010b) *An A–Z of the Genetic Factors in Autism: A Handbook for Professionals.* London: Jessica Kingsley Publishers.

Aitken, K.J. (2011) *Sleep Difficulties and Autism Spectrum Disorders.* London: Jessica Kingsley Publishers.

Aitken, K.J. (2012) *Sleep Difficulties and Autistic Spectrum Disorders: A Guide for Parents and Professionals.* London: Jessica Kingsley Publishers.

Ali, M., Auger, R.R., Slocumb, N.L. and Morgenthaler, T.I. (2009) 'Idiopathic hypersomnia: Clinical features and response to treatment.' *Journal of Clinical Sleep Medicine, 5*(6): 562–568.

Allen, K.D., Kuhn, B.R., DeHaai, K.A. and Wallace, D.P. (2013) 'Evaluation of a behavioral treatment package to reduce sleep problems in children with Angelman Syndrome.' *Research in Developmental Disabilities, 34*: 676–686.

Alloussi, S.H., Murtz, G., Lang, C. Madersbacher, H. *et al.* (2010) 'Desmopressin treatment regimens in monosymptomatic and nonmonosymptomatic enuresis: A review from a clinical perspective.' *Journal of Pediatric Urology, 7*(2): 10–20.

Alvarez-Arenal, A., Junquera, L.M., Fernandez, J.P., Gonzalez, I. and Olay, S. (2002) 'Effect of occlusal splint and transcutaneous electric nerve stimulation on the signs and symptoms of temporomandibular disorders in patients with bruxism.' *Journal of Oral Rehabilitation, 29*(9): 858–863.

American Academy of Sleep Medicine (2005) *International Classification of Sleep Disorders: Diagnostic and Coding Manual* (2nd edn). Westchester, IL: AASP.

American Academy of Sleep Medicine (2014) *International Classification of Sleep Disorders: Diagnostic and Coding Manual* (3rd end). Westchester, IL: AASP.

American Psychiatric Association (2013) *Diagnostic and Statistical Manual of Mental Disorders, Fifth Edition (DSM-5).* Arlington, VA: American Psychiatric Publishing.

Andersen, I.M., Kaczmarska, J., McGrew, S.G. and Malow, B.A. (2008) 'Melatonin for insomnia in children with autism spectrum disorders.' *Journal of Child Neurology, 23*(5): 482–485.

Anderson, B.M., Schnetz-Boutau, N.C., Bartlett, J., Wotawa, A.M. *et al.* (2009) 'Examination of association of genes in the serotonin system to autism.' *Neurogenetics, 10*(3): 209–216.

Anderson, J.R. and Meno, P. (2003) 'Psychological influences on yawning in children.' *Current Psychology Letters, 11*(2): 2–7.

Appleton, R.E., Jones, A.P., Gamble, C., Williamson, P.R., Wiggs, L., Montgomery, P., Sutcliffe, A., Barker, C. and Gringras, P. (2012) 'The use of melatonin in children with neurodevelopmental disorders and impaired sleep: A randomised, double-blind, placebo-controlled, parallel study (MENDS).' *Health Technology Assessment, 16*(40): i–239. doi: 10.3310/hta16400.

Aran, A., Einen, M., Lin, L., Plazzi, G. *et al.* (2010) 'Clinical and therapeutic aspects of childhood narcolepsy-cataplexy: A retrospective study of 51 children.' *Sleep, 33*(11): 1457–1464.

Arbuckle, R., Abetz, L., Durmer, J.S., Ivanenko, A. *et al.* (2010) 'Development of the Pediatric Restless Legs Syndrome Severity Scale (P-RLS-SS)©: A patient-reported outcome measure of pediatric RLS symptoms and impact.' *Sleep Medicine, 11*: 897–906.

Archer, S.N., Robilliard, D.L., Skene, D.J., Smits, M. *et al.* (2003) 'A length polymorphism in the circadian clock gene Per3 is linked to delayed sleep phase syndrome and extreme diurnal preference.' *Sleep, 26*(4): 413–415.

Armitage, R., Flynn, H., Hoffmann, R., Vazquez, D. *et al.* (2009) 'Early developmental changes in sleep in infants: The impact of maternal depression.' *Sleep, 32*: 693–696.

Ashbaugh, R. and Peck, S.M. (1998) 'Treatment of sleep problems in a toddler: A replication of the faded bedtime with response cost protocol.' *Journal of Applied Behaviour Analysis, 31*(1): 127–129.

Ashwood, P., Krakowiak, P., Hertz-Picciotto, I., Hansen, R. *et al.* (2011) 'Elevated plasma cytokines in autism spectrum disorders provide evidence 4 of immune dysfunction and are associated with impaired behavioral outcome.' *Brain, Behavior, and Immunity, 25*(1): 40–45. doi:10.1016/j.bbi.2010.08.003.

Ashwood, P., Kwong, C., Hansen, R., Hertz-Picciotto, I. *et al.* (2008) 'Brief report: plasma leptin levels are elevated in autism: Association with early onset phenotype?' *Journal of Autism and Developmental Disorders, 38*(1): 169–175.

Atsumi, T., Fujisawa, S., Nakabayashi, Y., Kawai, T., Yasui, T. and Yonosaki, K. (2004) 'Pleasant feeling from watching a comical video enhances free radical scavenging capacity in human whole saliva.' *Journal of Psychosomatic Research, 56:* 377–379.

Aurora, R.N., Zak, R.S., Auerbach, S.H., Casey, K.R. *et al.* (2010) 'Best practice guide for the treatment of nightmare disorder in adults.' *Journal of Clinical Sleep Medicine, 6*(4): 389–401.

Avidan, A.Y. and Chervin, R.D. (2002) 'ESS dot com.' *Sleep Medicine, 3*(5): 405–410.

Baglioni, C., Spiegelhalder, K., Lombardo, C. and Riemann, D. (2010) 'Sleep and emotions: A focus on insomnia.' *Sleep Medicine Reviews, 14*: 227–238.

Baird, J., Hill, C.M., Kendrick, T., Inskip, H.M. and the SWS Study Group (2009) 'Infant sleep disturbance is associated with preconceptional psychological distress: Findings from the Southampton Women's Survey.' *Sleep, 32*(4): 566–568.

Ball, H.L. (2003) 'Breastfeeding, bed-sharing, and infant sleep.' *Birth, 30*(3): 181–188.

Bamne, M.N., Mansour, H., Monk, T.H., Buysse, D.J. and Nimgaonkar, V.L. (2010) 'Approaches to unravel the genetics of sleep.' *Sleep Medicine Reviews, 14*(6): 397–404.

Banerjee, D., Vitiello, M.V. and Grunstein, R.R. (2004) 'Pharmacotherapy for excessive daytime sleepiness.' *Sleep Medicine Reviews, 8*(5): 339–354.

Barion, A. and Zee, P.C. (2007) 'A clinical approach to circadian rhythm sleep disorders.' *Sleep Medicine, 8*(6): 566–577.

Barnoy, E.L., Najdowski, A.C., Tarbox, J., Wilke, A.E. and Nollet, M.D. (2009) 'Evaluation of a multicomponent intervention for diurnal bruxism in a young child with autism.' *Journal of Applied Behavior Analysis, 42*(4): 845–848.

Basta, M., Lin, H-M., Pejovic, S., Sarrigiannidis, A. *et al.* (2008) 'Lack of regular exercise, depression, and degree of apnea are predictors of excessive daytime sleepiness in patients with sleep apnea: Sex differences.' *Journal of Clinical Sleep Medicine, 4*(1): 19–25.

Baxter, P. (ed.) (2001) *Vitamin Responsive Conditions in Paediatric Neurology.* London: MacKeith Press.

Bazil, C.W. (2003) 'Epilepsy and sleep disturbance.' *Epilepsy & Behavior, 4:* S39–S45.

Bazil, C.W. (2004) 'Nocturnal seizures.' *Seminars in Neurology, 24*(3): 293–300.

Bazil, C.W., Short, D.W., Crispin, D. and Zheng, W. (2000) 'Patients with intractable epilepsy have low melatonin, which increases following seizures.' *Neurology, 55:* 1746–1748.

Beebe, D.W. and Gozal, D. (2002) 'Obstructive sleep apnea and the prefrontal cortex: Towards a comprehensive model linking nocturnal upper airway obstruction to daytime cognitive and behavioral deficits.' *Journal of Sleep Research, 11*(1): 1–16.

Beenhakker, M.P. and Huguenard, J.R. (2009) 'Neurons that fire together also conspire together: Is normal sleep circuitry hijacked to generate epilepsy?' *Neuron, 62:* 612–632.

Ben-Menachem, E. (2007) 'Weight issues for people with epilepsy – a review.' *Epilepsia, 48*(s9): 42–45.

Benington, J.H. and Heller, H.C. (1995) 'Restoration of brain energy metabolism as the function of sleep.' *Progress in Neurobiology, 45:* 347–360.

Berlucchi, M., Salsi, D., Valetti, L., Parrinello, G. and Nicolai, P. (2007) 'The role of mometasone furoate aqueous nasal spray in the treatment of adenoidal hypertrophy in the pediatric age group: Preliminary results of a prospective, randomized study.' *Pediatrics, 119:* e1392–e1397.

Berman, S.M., Kuczenski, R., McCracken, J.T. and London, E.D. (2009) 'Potential adverse effects of amphetamine treatment on brain and behavior: A review.' *Molecular Psychiatry, 14*(2): 123–142.

Berthier, M.L., Santamaria, J., Encabo, H. and Tolosa, E.S. (1992) 'Recurrent hypersomnia in two adolescent males with Asperger's syndrome.' *Journal of the American Academy of Child & Adolescent Psychiatry, 31*(4): 735–738.

Billiard M., Guilleminault, C. and Dement, W.C. (1975) 'A menstruation-linked periodic hypersomnia: Kleine-Levin syndrome or new clinical entity?' *Neurology, 25:* 436–443.

Bixler, E.O., Vgontzas, A.N., Lin, H.M., Calhoun, S.L. *et al.* (2005) 'Excessive daytime sleepiness in a general population sample: The role of sleep apnea, age, obesity, diabetes, and depression.' *Journal of Clinical Endocrinology and Metabolism, 90*(8): 4510–4515.

Bjorvatn, B., Sagen, I.M., Oyane, N., Waage, S. *et al.* (2007) 'The association between sleep duration, body mass index and metabolic measures in the Hordaland Health Study.' *Journal of Sleep Research, 16:* 66–76.

Black, J. and Houghton, W.C. (2006) 'Sodium oxybate improves excessive daytime sleepiness in narcolepsy.' *Sleep, 29*(7): 939–946.

Blouin, A.M., Thannickal, T.C., Worley, P.F., Baraban, J.M. *et al.* (2005) 'Narp immunostaining of human hypocretin (orexin) neurons: Loss in narcolepsy.' *Neurology, 65:* 1189–1192.

Blunden, S., Lushington, K., Lorenzen, B., Ooi, T., Fung, F. and Kennedy, D. (2004) 'Are sleep problems under-recognised in general practice?' *Archives of Disease in Childhood, 89*: 708–712.

Boergers, J., Hart, C., Owens, J.A., Streisand, R. and Spirito, A. (2007) 'Child sleep disorders: Associations with parental sleep duration and daytime sleepiness.' *Journal of Family Psychology, 21*(1): 88–94.

Boeve, B.F. (2010) 'REM sleep behavior disorder: Updated review of the core features, the RBD-Neurodegenerative Disease Association, evolving concepts, controversies, and future directions.' *Annals of the New York Academy of Science, 1184*: 15–54.

Bollard, J. and Nettlebeck, T. (1982) 'A component analysis of dry-bed training for treatment of bedwetting.' *Behaviour Research and Therapy, 20*: 383–390.

Bonnet, C., Roubertie, A., Doummar, D., Bahi-Buisson, N. *et al.* (2010) 'Developmental and benign movement disorders in childhood.' *Movement Disorders, 25*(10): 1317–1334.

Braam, W., Didden, R., Smits, M.G. and Curfs, L.M. (2008) 'Melatonin for chronic insomnia in Angelman syndrome: A randomized placebo-controlled trial.' *Journal of Child Neurology, 23*(6): 649–654.

Braam, W., Smits, M.G., Didden, R., Korzilius, H. *et al.* (2009) 'Exogenous melatonin for sleep problems in individuals with intellectual disability: A meta-analysis.' *Developmental Medicine and Child Neurology, 51*(5): 340–349.

Braam, W., van Geijlswijk, I., Keijzer, H., Smits, M.G. *et al.* (2010) 'Loss of response to melatonin treatment is associated with slow melatonin metabolism.' *Journal of Intellectual Disability Research, 54*(6): 547–555.

Brosnan, M., Turner-Cobb, J., Munro-Naan, Z. and Jessop, D. (2009) 'Absence of a normal cortisol awakening response (CAR) in adolescent males with Asperger syndrome.' *Psychoneuroendocrinology, 34*(7): 1095–1100.

Brown, C.M. and Austin D.W. (2009) 'Commentary: Fatty acids, breastfeeding and autism spectrum disorder.' *Electronic Journal of Applied Psychology: Innovations in Autism, 5*(1): 49–52.

Bruni, O., Ferri, R., Vittori, E., Novelli, L. *et al.* (2007) 'Sleep architecture and NREM alterations in children and adolescents with Asperger syndrome.' *Sleep, 30*(11): 1577–1585.

Bruni, O., Ottaviano, S., Guidetti, V., Romoli, M. *et al.* (1996) 'The Sleep Disturbance Scale for Children (SDSC): Construction and validation of an instrument to evaluate sleep disturbances in childhood and adolescence.' *Journal of Sleep Research, 5*(4): 251–261.

Bruni, O., Verrillo, E., Novelli, L. and Ferri, R. (2010) 'Prader-Willi syndrome: Sorting out the relationships between obesity, hypersomnia, and sleep apnea.' *Current Opinion in Pulmonary Medicine, 16*(6): 568–573.

Buckley, A.W., Rodriguez, A.J., Jennison, K., Buckley, J. *et al.* (2010) 'Rapid eye movement sleep percentage in children with autism compared with children with developmental delay and typical development.' *Archives of Pediatric and Adolescent Medicine, 164*(11): 1032–1037.

Budhiraja, R. (2007) 'The man who fought in sleep.' *Journal of Clinical Sleep Medicine, 3*(4): 427–428.

Burgess, M., Marks, I.M. and Gill, M. (1994) 'Postal self-exposure treatment of recurrent nightmares.' *British Journal of Psychiatry, 165*(3): 388–391.

Burke, R.V., Kuhn, B.R. and Peterson, J.L. (2004) 'Brief report: A "storybook" ending to children's bedtime problems – the use of a rewarding social story to reduce bedtime resistance and frequent night waking.' *Journal of Pediatric Psychology, 29*(5): 389–396.

Burlina, A.B., Burlina, A.P., Hyland, K., Bonafe, L. and Blau, N. (2001) 'Autistic syndrome and aromatic L-amino acid decarboxylase deficiency.' *Journal of Inherited Metabolic Disease, 24*(Suppl 1): 34.

Butler, R.J., Golding, J., Northstone, K. and Study Team ALSPAC (2005) 'Nocturnal enuresis at 7.5 years old: Prevalence and analysis of clinical signs.' *British Journal of Urology International, 96*: 404–410.

Buysse, D.J., Reynolds, C.F., Monk, T.H., Berman, S.R. and Kupfer, D.J. (1989) 'The Pittsburgh Sleep Quality Index (PSQI): A new instrument for psychiatric research and practice.' *Psychiatry Research, 28*: 193–213.

Byars, A.W., Byars, K.C., Johnson, C.S., deGrauw, T.J. *et al.* (2008) 'The relationship between sleep problems and neuropsychological functioning in children with first recognized seizures.' *Epilepsy and Behavior, 13*(4): 607–613.

Cain, N. and Gradisar, M. (2010) 'Electronic media use and sleep in school-aged children and adolescents: A review.' *Sleep Medicine, 11*: 735–742.

Caione, P., Arena, F., Biraghi, M., Cigna, R.M. *et al.* (1997) 'Nocturnal enuresis and daytime wetting: A multicentric trial with oxybutynin and desmopressin.' *European Urology, 31*(4): 459–463.

Calandre, L., Martinez-Martin, P. and Campos-Castellano, J. (1978) 'Tratamiento del syndrome de Lennox con trigliceridos de cadena media.' *Anales Espanoles de Pediatria, 11*: 189–194.

Camfield, P. and Camfield C. (2002) 'Epileptic syndromes in childhood: Clinical features, outcomes, and treatment.' *Epilepsia, 43*(Suppl 3): 27–32.

Camfield, P., Gordon, K., Dooley, J. and Camfield, C. (1996) 'Melatonin appears ineffective in children with intellectual deficits and fragmented sleep: six "N of 1" trials.' *Journal of Child Neurology, 11*: 341–343.

Canitano, R. (2007) 'Epilepsy in autism spectrum disorders.' *European Journal of Child and Adolescent Psychiatry, 16*(1): 61–66.

Capdevila, O.S., Kheirandish-Gozal, L., Dayyat, E. and Gozal, D. (2008) 'Pediatric obstructive sleep apnea complications, management, and long-term outcomes.' *Proceedings of the American Thoracic Society, 5*: 274–282.

Carpenter, J.S. and Andrykowski, M.A. (1998) 'Psychometric evaluation of the Pittsburgh Sleep Quality Index.' *Journal of Psychosomatic Research, 45*(1): 5–13.

Carrasco, M., Volkmar, F.R. and Bloch, M.H. (2012) 'Pharmacologic treatment of repetitive behaviors in autism spectrum disorders: Evidence of publication bias.' *Pediatrics, 129*(5): e1301–1310. doi: 10.1542/peds.2011-3285.

Carskadon, M.A., Dement, W.C., Mittler, M.M., Roth, T. *et al.* (1986) 'Guidelines for the Multiple Sleep Latency Test (MSLT): A standard measure of sleepiness.' *Sleep, 9*: 519–524.

Carvalho, F.R., Lentini-Oliveira, D., Machado, M.A., Prado, G.F., Prado, L.B. and Saconato, H. (2007) 'Oral appliances and functional orthopaedic appliances for obstructive sleep apnoea in children.' *Cochrane Database of Systematic Reviews, Issue 4*(2): CD005520.

Casella, E.B., Valente, M., Navarro, J.M. and Kok, F. (2005) 'Vitamin B12 deficiency in infancy as a cause of developmental regression.' *Brain and Development, 27*(8): 592–594.

Casey, B.J., Duhoux, S. and Cohen, M.W. (2010) 'Adolescence: What do transmission, transition, and translation have to do with it?' *Neuron, 67*: 749–760.

Casez, O., Dananchet, Y. and Besson, G. (2005) 'Migraine and somnambulism.' *Neurology, 65*: 1334–1335.

Cassisi, J.E., McGlynn, F.D. and Belles, D.R. (1987) 'EMG-activated feedback alarms for the treatment of nocturnal bruxism: Current status and future directions.' *Biofeedback and Self Regulation, 12*(1): 13–30.

Castriotta, R.J., Atanasov, S., Mark C. Wilde, M.C., Masel, B.E. et al. (2009) 'Treatment of sleep disorders after traumatic brain injury.' *Journal of Clinical Sleep Medicine, 5*(2): 137–144.

Challamel, M.J., Mazzola, M.E., Nevsimalova, S., Cannard, C. *et al.* (1994) 'Narcolepsy in children.' *Sleep, 17*(Suppl 8): S17–20.

Chaste, P., Clement, N., Mercati, O., Guillaume, J.L. *et al.* (2010) 'Identification of pathway-biased and deleterious melatonin receptor mutants in autism spectrum disorders and in the general population.' *PloS One, 5*(7): e11495.

Chervin, R.D., Hedger, K., Dillon, J.E. and Pituch, K.J. (2000) 'Pediatric Sleep Questionnaire (PSQ): Validity and reliability of scales for sleep-disordered breathing, snoring, sleepiness, and behavioral problems.' *Sleep Medicine, 1*: 21–32.

Chervin, R.D., Ruzicka, D.L., Giordani, B.J., Weatherly, R.A. *et al.* (2006) 'Sleep-disordered breathing, behavior, and cognition in children before and after adenotonsillectomy.' *Pediatrics, 117*(4): e769–778.

Cheyne, J.A. and Girard, T.A. (2009) 'The body unbound: Vestibular-motor hallucinations and out-of-body experiences.' *Cortex, 45*(2): 201–215.

Chez, M.G., Buchanan, T., Aimonovitch, M., Mrazek, S. *et al.* (2004) Frequency of EEG abnormalities in age-matched siblings of autistic children with abnormal sleep EEG patterns.' *Epilepsy and Behavior, 5*: 159–162.

Chez, M.G., Chang, M., Krasne, V., Coughlan, C., Kominsky, M. and Schwartz, A. (2006) 'Frequency of epileptiform EEG abnormalities in a sequential screening of autistic patients with no known clinical epilepsy from 1996 to 2005.' *Epilepsy and Behavior, 8*: 267–271.

Chirakalwasan, N., Hassan, F., Kaplish, N., Fetterolf, J. and Chervin, R.D. (2009) 'Near resolution of sleep related rhythmic movement disorder after CPAP for OSA.' *Sleep Medicine, 10*: 497–500.

Chiu, Y.H., Chen, C.H. and Shen, W.W. (2008) 'Somnambulism secondary to olanzapine treatment in one patient with bipolar disorder.' *Progress in Neuropsychopharmacology and Biological Psychiatry, 32*: 581–582.

Coleman, M. and Gillberg, C. (2011) *The Autisms.* Oxford: Oxford University Press.

Colles, S.L., Dixon, J.B. and O'Brien, P.E. (2007) 'Night eating syndrome and nocturnal snacking: Association with obesity, binge eating and psychological distress.' *International Journal of Obesity (London), 31*(11): 1722–1730.

Conway, S.G., Castro, L., Lopes-Conceicao, M.C., Hachui, H. and Tufic, S. (2011) 'Psychological treatment for sleepwalking: Two case reports.' *Clinics (Sao Paulo), 66*(3): 517–520.

Coon, H., Dunn, D., Lainhart, J., Miller, J. *et al.* (2005) 'Possible association between autism and variants in the brain-expressed tryptophan hydroxylase gene (TPH2).' *American Journal of Medical Genetics B, 135*(1): 42–46.

Corkum, P., Panton, R., Ironside, S., Macpherson, M., Williams, T. (2008). 'Acute impact of immediate release methylphenidate administered three times a day on sleep in children with attention deficit/ hyperactivity disorder.' *Journal of Pediatric Psychology, 33*(4): 368–379.

Cortese, S., Konofal, E. and Yateman, N. (2006) 'Sleep and alertness in children with attention deficit hyperactivity disorder: A systematic review of the literature.' *Sleep, 29*: 504–511.

Cotton, S. and Richdale, A. (2006) 'Brief report: Parental descriptions of sleep problems in children with autism, Down syndrome, and Prader-Willi syndrome.' *Research in Developmental Disabilities, 27*(2): 151–161.

Cotton, S. and Richdale, A. (2010) 'Sleep patterns and behaviour in typically developing children and children with autism, Down syndrome, Prader-Willi syndrome and intellectual disability.' *Research in Autism Disorders, 4*(3): 490–500.

Coutinho, A.M., Oliveira, G., Morgadinho, T., Fesel, C. *et al.* (2004) 'Variants of the serotonin transporter gene (SLC6A4) significantly contribute to hyperserotonemia in autism.' *Molecular Psychiatry, 9*(3): 264–271.

Coutinho, A.M., Sousa, I., Martins, M., Correia, C. *et al.* (2007) 'Evidence for epistasis between SLC6A4 and ITGB3 in autism etiology and in the determination of platelet serotonin levels.' *Human Genetics, 121*(2): 243–256.

Crabtree, V.McL., Ivanenko, A., O'Brien, L.M. and Gozal, D. (2003) 'Periodic limb movement disorder of sleep in children.' *Journal of Sleep Research, 12*: 73–81.

Crick, F. and Mitchison, G. (1983) 'The function of dream sleep.' *Nature, 304*: 111–114.

Dahl, R.E., Holttum, J. and Trubnick, L. (1994) 'A clinical picture of child and adolescent narcolepsy.' *Journal of the American Academy of Child and Adolescent Psychiatry, 33*(6): 834–841.

Daley, M., Morin, C.M., LeBlanc, M., Gregoire, J.P. and Savoir, J. (2009) 'The economic burden of insomnia: Direct and indirect costs for individuals with insomnia syndrome, insomnia symptoms, and good sleepers.' *Sleep, 32*(1): 55–64.

Dauvilliers, Y., Baumann, C.R., Carlander, B. Bischof, M. *et al.* (2003) 'CSF hypocretin-1 levels in narcolepsy, Kleine-Levin syndrome, and other hypersomnias and neurological conditions.' *Journal of Neurology, Neurosurgery and Psychiatry, 74*: 1667–1673.

Dauvilliers, Y., Rompré, S., Gagnon, J-F. and Vendette, M. (2007) 'REM sleep characteristics in narcolepsy and REM sleep behavior disorder.' *Sleep, 30*(7): 844–849.

Davé, S., Sherr, L., Senior, R. and Nazareth, I. (2009) 'Major paternal depression and child consultation for developmental and behavioural problems.' *British Journal of General Practice, 59*: 180–185.

Davis, B.J., Rajput, A., Rajput, M.L., Aul, E.A. and Eichorn, G.R. (2000) 'A randomized, double-blind placebo-controlled trial of iron in restless legs syndrome.' *European Neurology, 43*: 70–75.

Davis, C.L., Tkacz, J., Gregoski, M., Boyle, C.A. and Lovrekovic, G. (2006) 'Aerobic exercise and snoring in overweight children: A randomized controlled trial.' *Obesity (Silver Spring), 14*(11): 1985–1991.

Davis, C.L., Tomporowski, P.D., Boyle, C.A., Waller, J.L. *et al.* (2007) 'Effects of aerobic exercise on overweight children's cognitive functioning: A randomized controlled trial.' *Research Quarterly in Exercise and Sport, 78*(5): 510–519.

De Leersnyder, H., Claustrat, B., Munnich, A. and Verloes, A. (2006) 'Circadian rhythm disorder in a rare disease: Smith-Magenis syndrome.' *Molecular and Cellular Endocrinology, 252*(1–2): 88–91.

DeMore, M., Cataldo, M., Tierney, E. and Slifer, K. (2009) 'Behavioral approaches to training developmentally disabled children for an overnight EEG procedure.' *Journal of Developmental and Physical Disability, 21*(4): 245–251.

Denne, S.C. (2012) 'Pediatric clinical trial registration and trial results: An urgent need for improvement.' *Pediatrics, 129*(5): e1320–1321. doi:10.1542/peds.2012-0621.

De Wachter, S., Vernmandel, A., de Moerloose, K. and Wyndaele, J.J. (2002) 'Value of increase in bladder capacity in treatment of refractory monosymptomatic nocturnal eneuresis in children.' *Urology, 60*: 1090–1094.

Didden, R., Curfs, L.M., van Driel, S. and de Moor, J.M. (2002) 'Sleep problems in children and young adults with developmental disabilities: Home-based functional assessment and treatment.' *Journal of Behavior Therapy and Experimental Psychiatry, 33*(1): 49–58.

Diomedi, M., Curatolo, P., Scalise, A., Placidia, F., Caretto, F. and Gigli, G.L. (1999) 'Sleep abnormalities in mentally retarded autistic subjects: Down's syndrome with mental retardation and normal subjects.' *Brain & Development, 21*: 548–553.

Dominick, K.. Davis, N.O., Lainhart, J., Tager-Flusberg, H. and Folstein, S. (2007) 'Atypical behaviors in children with autism and children with a history of language impairment.' *Research in Developmental Disabilities, 28*(2): 145–162.

Donlea, J.M. and Shaw, P.J. (2009) 'Sleeping together: Using social interactions to understand the role of sleep in plasticity.' *Advances in Genetics, 68*: 57–81.

Doo, S. and Wing, Y.K.(2006) 'Sleep problems of children with pervasive developmental disorders: Correlation with parental stress.' *Developmental Medicine and Child Neurology, 48*: 650–655.

Dosman, C.F., Brian, J.A., Drmic, I.E., Senthilselvan, A. *et al.* (2007) 'Children With autism: Effect of iron supplementation on sleep and ferritin.' *Pediatric Neurology, 36*: 152–158.

Dosman, C., Drmic, I., Brian, J., Senthilselvan, A. *et al.* (2006) 'Ferritin as an indicator of suspected iron deficiency in children with autism spectrum disorder: Prevalence of low serum ferritin concentration. *Developmental Medicine and Child Neurology, 48*: 1008–1009.

Drake, C., Nickel, C., Burduvali, E., Roth, T., Jeffereson, C. and Pietro, B. (2003) 'The Pediatric Daytime Sleepiness Scale (PDSS): Sleep habits and school outcomes in middle-school children.' *Sleep, 26*(4): 455–458.

Dunn, W. (1999) *Sensory profile.* New York, NY: Harcourt Assessment Inc.

Droogleever Fortuyn, H.A., Swinkels, S., Buitelaar, J., Renier, W.O. *et al.* (2008) 'High prevalence of eating disorders in narcolepsy with cataplexy: A case-control study.' *Sleep, 31*(3): 335–341.

Earley, C.J., Allen, R.P., Beard, J.L. and Connor, J.R. (2000) 'Insight into the pathophysiology of restless legs syndrome.' *Journal of Neuroscience Research, 62*: 623–628.

Ebisawa, T. (2007) 'Circadian rhythms in the CNS and peripheral clock disorders: Human sleep disorders and clock genes.' *Journal of Pharmacological Science, 103*: 150–154.

Edwards, S.D. and van der Spuy, H.I. (1985) 'Hypnotherapy as a treatment for enuresis.' *Journal of Child Psychology Psychiatry & Allied Disciplines, 26*(1): 161–170.

Elkhayat, H.A., Hassanein, S.M., Tomoum, H.Y., Abd-Elhamid, I.A. *et al.* (2010) 'Melatonin and sleep-related problems in children with intractable epilepsy.' *Pediatric Neurology, 42*(4): 249–254.

Erichsen, D., Ferri, R. and Gozal D. (2010) 'Ropinirole in restless legs syndrome and periodic limb movement disorder.' *Therapeutics and Clinical Risk Management, 6*: 173–182.

Espie, C.A. and Kyle, S.D. (2009) 'Primary insomnia: An overview of practical management using cognitive behavioral techniques.' *Sleep Medicine Clinics, 4*: 559–569.

Evans, J.H.C. (2001) 'Evidence based paediatrics: Evidence based management of nocturnal enuresis.' *British Medical Journal, 323*: 1167–1169.

Faraone, S.V., Glatt, S.J., Bukstein, O.G., Lopez, F.A. *et al.* (2009) 'Effects of once-daily oral and transdermal methylphenidate on sleep behavior of children with ADHD.' *Journal of Attention Disorders, 12*(4): 308–315.

Fass, R., Quan, S.F., O'Connor, G.T., Ervin, A. and Iber, C. (2005) 'Predictors of heartburn during sleep in a large prospective cohort study.' *Chest, 127*(5): 1658–1666.

Fauteck, J.D., Schmidt, H., Lerchl, A., Kurlemann, G. and Wittkowski, W. (1999) 'Melatonin in epilepsy: First results of replacement therapy and first clinical results.' *Biological Signals and Receptors, 8*: 105–110.

Ferrara, M., Moroni, F., De Gennaro, L. and Nobili, L. (2012) 'Hippocampal sleep features: Relations to human memory function.' *Frontiers in Neurology, 3*(57): 1–9. doi: 10.3389/fneur.2012.00057.

Fielding, D. (1980) 'The response of day and night wetting children and children who wet only at night to retention control training and the eneuresis alarm.' *Behaviour Research and Therapy, 18*: 305–317.

Fifer, W.P., Byrd, D.L., Kaku, M., Eigsti, I-M. *et al.* (2010) "Newborn infants learn during sleep.' *Proceedings of the National Academy of Science USA, 107*(22): 10320–10323.

Findley, L., Unverzagt, M., Guchu, R., Fabrizio, M. *et al.* (1995) 'Vigilance and automobile accidents in patients with sleep apnea or narcolepsy.' *Chest, 108*: 619–624.

Fisher, C., Kahn, E., Edwards, A. and Davis, D.M.(1973) 'A psychological study of nightmares and night terrors: The suppression of stage 4 night terrors with diazepam.' *Archives of General Psychiatry, 28*: 252–259.

Fitzgerald, M.P., Thom, D.H., Wassel-Fyr, C., Subak, L. *et al.* (2006) 'Childhood urinary symptoms predict adult overactive bladder symptoms.' *Journal of Urology, 175*(3 Pt 1): 989–993.

Flanagan, O.J. (2001) *Dreaming Souls: Sleep, Dreams and the Evolution of the Conscious Mind.* New York, NY: Oxford University Press.

Ford, D.E. and Kamerow, D.B. (1989) 'Epidemiologic study of sleep disturbances and psychiatric disorders. An opportunity for prevention?' *Journal of the American Medical Association, 262*(11): 1479–1484.

Fox, N.A. (2007) 'Insufficient evidence to confirm effectiveness of oral appliances in treatment of obstructive sleep apnoea syndrome in children.' *Evidence Based Dentistry, 8*(3): 84.

France, K.G. and Hudson S.M. (1990) Behavioral management of infant sleep disturbance.' *Journal of Applied Behavior Analysis, 23*: 91–98.

Francis, R.C. (2011) *The Ultimate Muystery of Inheritance: Epigenetics.* New York, NY: Norton & Co.

Frauscher, B., Gschliesser, V., Brandauer, E., Marti, I. *et al.* (2010) 'REM sleep behavior disorder in 703 sleep-disorder patients: The importance of eliciting a comprehensive sleep history.' *Sleep Medicine, 11*: 167–171.

Friedman, A. and Luiselli, J.K. (2008) 'Excessive daytime sleep: Behavioral assessment and intervention in a child with autism.' *Behavior Modification, 32*(4): 548–555.

Friedman, A.G. and Ollendick, T.H. (1989) 'Treatment programs for severe night-time fears: A methodological note.' *Journal of Behavior Therapy and Experimental Psychiatry, 20*(2): 171–178.

Friman, P.C., Hoff, K.E., Schnoes, C., Freeman, K.A. *et al.* (1999) 'The bedtime pass: An approach to bedtime crying and leaving the room.' *Archives of Pediatric and Adolescent Medicine, 153*(10): 1027–1029.

Gagnon, J-F., Postuma, R.B. and Montplaisir, J. (2006) 'Update on the pharmacology of REM sleep behavior disorder.' *Neurology, 67*: 742–747.

Gagnon, Y., Mayer, P., Morisson, F., Rompré, P.H. *et al.* (2004) 'Aggravation of respiratory disturbances by the use of an occlusal splint in apneic patients: A pilot study.' *International Journal of Prosthodontics, 17*: 447–453.

Garcia-Borreguero, D. and Williams, A.M. (2010) 'Dopaminergic augmentation of restless legs syndrome.' *Sleep Medicine Reviews, 14*(5): 339–346.

Garcia-Fernàndez, J. (2005) 'The genesis and evolution of homeobox gene clusters.' *Nature Reviews: Genetics, 6*(12): 881–892.

Garstang, J. and Wallis, M. (2006) 'Randomized controlled trial of melatonin for children with autistic spectrum disorders and sleep problems.' *Child Care Health and Development, 32*(5): 585–589.

Gau, S.S-F. and Chiang, H-L. (2009) 'Sleep problems and disorders among adolescents with persistent and subthreshold attention-deficit/hyperactivity disorders.' *Sleep, 32*(5): 671–679.

Gelineau, J. (1880) 'De la narcolepsie.' Gazette Hopital (Paris), 53: 626–628.

Geschwind, D.H. and Levitt, P. (2007) 'Autism spectrum disorders: Developmental disconnection syndromes.' *Current Opinion in Neurobiology, 17*: 103–111.

Giannotti, F., Cortesi, F., Cerquiglini A., Miraglia, D. *et al.* (2008) 'An investigation of sleep characteristics, EEG abnormalities and epilepsy in developmentally regressed and non-regressed children with autism.' *Journal of Autism and Developmental Disorders, 38*: 1888–1897.

Gibson, E.S., Powles, A.C.P. Thabane, L., O'Brien, S. *et al.* (2006) '"Sleepiness" is serious in adolescence: Two surveys of 3235 Canadian students.' *BMC Public Health, 6*: 116. doi:10.1186/1471-2458-6-116.

Glazener, C.M.A. and Evans, J.H.C. (2002) 'Desmopressin for nocturnal enuresis in children.' *Cochrane Database of Systematic Reviews, Issue 3.* Art. No.: CD002112. doi: 10.1002/14651858.CD002112.

Glazener, C.M.A. and Evans, J.H.C. (2004) 'Simple behavioural and physical interventions for nocturnal enuresis in children.' *Cochrane Database of Systematic Reviews, 2*: Art. No.: CD003637. doi: 10.1002/14651858.CD003637.pub2.

Glazener, C.M.A., Evans, J.H.C. and Cheuk, D.K.L. (2005) 'Complementary and miscellaneous interventions for nocturnal enuresis in children.' *Cochrane Database of Systematic Reviews, Issue 2.* Art. No.: CD005230. doi: 10.1002/14651858. CD005230.

Glazener, C.M.A., Evans, J.H.C. and Peto, R.E. (2003a) 'Tricyclic and related drugs for nocturnal enuresis in children.' *Cochrane Database of Systematic Reviews, Issue 3*: Art. No.: CD002117. doi: 10.1002/14651858.CD002117.

Glazener, C.M.A., Evans, J.H.C. and Peto, R.E. (2003b) 'Drugs for nocturnal enuresis in children (other than desmopressin and tricyclics).' *Cochrane Database of Systematic Reviews, Issue 4.* Art. No.: CD002238. doi: 10.1002/14651858.CD002238.

Glazener, C.M.A., Evans, J.H.C. and Peto, R.E. (2004) 'Complex behavioural and educational interventions for nocturnal enuresis in children.' *Cochrane Database of Systematic Reviews, Issue 1.* Art. No.: CD004668. doi: 10.1002/14651858. CD004668.

Glazener, C.M.A., Evans, J.H.C. and Peto, R.E. (2005) 'Alarm interventions for nocturnal enuresis in children.' *Cochrane Database of Systematic Reviews , Issue 1.* Art. No.: CD002911. doi: 10.1002/14651858.CD002911.

Glickman, G. (2010) 'Circadian rhythms and sleep in children with autism.' *Neuroscience and Biobehavioral Reviews, 34*: 755–768.

Glotzbach, S.F., Edgar, D.M. and Ariagno, R.L. (1995) 'Biological rhythmicity in preterm infants prior to discharge from neonatal intensive care.' *Pediatrics, 95*(2): 231–237.

Goldstein, D., Hahn, C.S., Hasher, L., Wiprzycka, U.J. and Zelazo, P.D. (2007) 'Time of day, intellectual performance, and behavioral problems in morning versus evening type adolescents: Is there a synchrony effect?' *Personality and Individual Differences, 42*(3): 431–440.

Goodlin-Jones, B.L., Sitnick, S.L., Tang, K., Liu, J. and Anders, T.F. (2008) 'The children's sleep habits questionnaire in toddlers and preschool children.' *Journal of Developmental and Behavioral Pediatrics, 9*(2): 82–88.

Gozal, D. (2008) 'Obstructive sleep apnea in children: Implications for the developing central nervous system.' *Seminars in Pediatric Neurology, 15*(2): 100–106.

Gozal, D., Kheirandish-Gozal, L., Capdevila, O.S., Dayyat, E. and Kheirandish, E. (2008) 'Prevalence of recurrent otitis media in habitually snoring school-aged children.' *Sleep Medicine, 9*(5): 549–554.

Gradisar, M., Lack, L., Richards, H., Harris, J. *et al.* (2007) 'The Flinders Fatigue Scale: Preliminary psychometric properties and clinical sensitivity of a new scale for measuring daytime fatigue associated with insomnia.' *Journal of Clinical Sleep Medicine, 3*(7): 722–728.

Gray, C.A. and Garand, J.D. (1993) 'Teaching children with autism to "read" social situations.' In: K.Quill (ed.) *Teaching Children with Autism: Strategies to Enhance Communication and Socialization.* New York, NY: Delmar.

Graziano, A.M. and Mooney, K.C. (1982) 'Behavioral treatment of "nightfears" in children: Maintenance of improvement at 2½- to 3-year follow-up.' *Journal of Consulting and Clinical Psychology, 50*(4): 598–599.

Gregory, A.M., Rijsdijk, F.V., Lau, J.Y.F., Dahl, R.E. and Eley, T.C. (2009) 'The direction of longitudinal associations between sleep problems and depression symptoms: A study of twins aged 8 and 10 years.' *Sleep, 32*(2): 189–199.

Gringras, P., Jones, A.P., Wiggs, L., Williamson, P.R. *et al.* (2012) 'Melatonin for sleep problems in children with neurodevelopmental disorders: Randomised double masked placebo controlled trial.' *British Medical Journal, 345*: e6664. doi: 10.1136/bmj.e6664.

Gruber, R., Sadeh, A. and Raviv, A. (2000) 'Instability of sleep patterns in children with attention-deficit/hyperactivity disorder.' *Journal of the American Academy of Child and Adolescent Psychiatry, 39*: 495–501.

Grundy, S.M., Brewer Jr, H.B., Cleeman, J.I., Smith Jr, S.C. *et al.* (2004) 'Definition of metabolic syndrome: Report of the National Heart, Lung, and Blood Institute/American Heart Association Conference on Scientific Issues Related to Definition.' *Circulation, 109*: 433–438.

Guilleminault, C., Cathala, J.P. and Castaigne, P. (1973) 'Effects of 5-hydroxytryptophan on sleep of a patient with brain-stem lesion.' *Electroencephalography and Clinical Neurophysiology, 34*: 177–184.

Guilleminault, C., Hagen, C.C. and Khaja, A.M. (2008) 'Catathrenia: Parasomnia or uncommon feature of sleep disordered breathing?' *Sleep, 31*(1): 132–139.

Gujar, N., Yoo, S-S., Hu, P. and Walker, M.P. (2010) 'The unrested resting brain: Sleep deprivation alters activity within the default-mode network.' *Journal of Cognitive Neuroscience, 22*(8): 1637–1648.

Halbower, A.C., McGinley, B.M. and Smith P.L. (2008) 'Treatment alternatives for sleep-disordered breathing in the pediatric population.' *Current Opinion in Pulmonary Medicine, 14*(6): 551–558.

Haldane, J.B.S. (1927) 'What Hot Means.' In: J.M.Smith (ed.) (1985) *On Being the Right Size and Other Essays.* Oxford: Oxford University Press.

Hallböök, T., Lundgren, J. and Rosén, I. (2007) 'Ketogenic diet improves sleep quality in children with therapy-resistant epilepsy.' *Epilepsia, 48*(1): 59–65.

Hallowell, L.M., Stewart, S.E., de Amortim E Silva, C.T. and Ditchfield, M.R. (2008) 'Reviewing the process of preparing children for MRI.' *Pediatric Radiology, 38*(3): 271–279.

Halpern, A., Mancini, M.C., Magalhães, M.E.C., Fisberg, M. *et al.* (2010) 'Metabolic syndrome, dyslipidemia, hypertension and type 2 diabetes in youth: From diagnosis to treatment.' *Diabetology & Metabolic Syndrome, 2*: 55.

Harris, L.S. and Purohit, A.P. (1977) 'Bladder training and eneuresis: A controlled trial.' *Behaviour Research and Therapy, 15*: 485–490.

Harris, M. and Grunstein, R.R. (2009) 'Treatments for somnambulism in adults: Assessing the evidence.' *Sleep Medicine Reviews, 13*(4): 295–297.

Harsh, J.R., Easley, A. and LeBourgeois, M.K. (2002) 'A measure of sleep hygiene.' *Sleep, 25*: A316.

Harvey, A.G., Murray, G., Chandler, R.A. and Soehner, A. (2010) 'Sleep disturbance as transdiagnostic: Consideration of neurobiological mechanisms.' *Clinical Psychology Review, 31*(2): 225–235.

Hasler, B. and Germain, A. (2009) 'Correlates and treatments of nightmares in adults.' *Sleep Medicine Clinics, 4*(4): 507–517.

Hayashi, E. (2001) 'Seasonal changes in sleep and behavioral problems in a pubescent case with autism.' *Psychiatry and Clinical Neurosciences, 55*(3): 223–224.

Henderson, J. and Jordan, S.S. (2010) 'Development and preliminary evaluation of the Bedtime Routines Questionnaire.' *Journal of Psychopathology and Behavioral Assessment, 32*: 271–280.

Henriksen, N. and Peterson, S. (2013) 'Behavioral treatment of bedwetting in an adolescent with autism.' *Journal of Developmental and Physical Disabilities, 25*(3): 313–323.

Herr, J.R. (2003) 'Letter to the editor: Re: autism–ear infections–glue ear–sleep disorders.' *Journal of Autism and Developmental Disorders, 33*(5): 557.

Heussler, H., Harris, D., Cooper, C., Dakin, S., Suresh, S. and Williams, G. (2008) 'Hypersomnolence in Prader Willi syndrome.' *Journal of Intellectual Disability Research, 52*(10): 814.

Hill, C.M., Hogan, A.M. and Karmiloff-Smith, A. (2007) 'To sleep, perchance to enrich learning?' *Archives of Disease in Childhood, 92*: 637–643.

Hiscock, H. and Wake, M. (2002) 'Randomised controlled trial of behavioural infant sleep intervention to improve infant sleep and maternal mood.' *British Medical Journal, 324*: 1062–1068.

Hoban, T. (2003) 'Rhythmic movement disorder in children.' *CNS Spectrums, 8*(2): 135–138.

Hobson, J.A. (2009) 'REM sleep and dreaming: Towards a theory of protoconsciousness.' *Nature Reviews: Neuroscience, 10*: 803–813.

Hobson, R.P. and Bishop, M. (2003) 'The pathogenesis of autism: Insights from congenital blindness.' *Philosophical Transactions of the Royal Society of London, Series B, 358*: 335–344.

Hobson, J.A. and McCarley, R. (1977) 'The brain as a dream state generator: An activation-synthesis hypothesis of the dream process.' *American Journal of Psychiatry, 134*: 1335–1348.

Hoffman C.D., Sweeney, D.P., Lopez-Wagner, M.C., Hodge, D. *et al.* (2008) 'Children with autism: Sleep problems and mothers' stress.' *Focus on Autism and Other Developmental Disabilities, 23*(3): 155–165.

Hofstra, W.A. and W. de Weerd, A. (2009) 'The circadian rhythm and its interaction with human epilepsy: A review of literature.' *Sleep Medicine Reviews, 13*: 413–420.

Högl, B., Oertel, W.H., Stiasny-Kolster, K., Geisler, P. *et al.* (2010) 'Treatment of moderate to severe restless legs syndrome: 2-year safety and efficacy of rotigotine transdermal patch.' *BMC Neurology, 10*: 86. doi:10.1186/1471-2377-10-86.

Holland, P.W.H., Booth, H.A.F. and Bruford, E.A. (2007) 'Classification and nomenclature of all human homeobox genes.' *BMC Biology, 5*: 47. doi:10.1186/1741-7007-5-47.

Hollinger, P., Khatami, R., Gugger, M., Hess, C.W. and Bassetti, C.L. (2006) 'Epilepsy and obstructive sleep apnea.' *European Neurology, 55*(2): 74–79.

Hoque, R. and Chesson Jr, A.L. (2009) 'Zolpidem-induced sleepwalking, sleep related eating disorder, and sleep-driving: Fluorine-18-flourodeoxyglucose positron emission tomography analysis, and a literature review of other unexpected clinical effects of Zolpidem.' *Journal of Clinical Sleep Medicine, 5*(5): 471–476.

Horvath, K., Papadimitriou, J.C., Rabsztyn, A., Drachenberg, C. and Tildon, J.T. (1999) 'Gastrointestinal abnormalities in children with autistic disorder.' *Journal of Pediatrics, 135*(5): 598–563.

Howell, M.J., Schenck, C.H. and Crow, S.J. (2009) 'A review of nighttime eating disorders.' *Sleep Medicine Reviews, 13*(1): 23–34.

Hu, V.W., Sarachana, T., Kim, K.S., Nguyen, A-T. *et al.* (2009) 'Gene expression profiling differentiates autism case–controls and phenotypic variants of autism spectrum disorders: Evidence for circadian rhythm dysfunction in severe autism.' *Autism Research, 2*(2): 78–97.

Hublin, C., Kaprio, J., Partinen, M., Heikkilä, K. and Koskenvuo, M. (1997) 'Prevalence and genetics of sleepwalking: A population based twin study.' *Neurology, 48*(1): 177–181.

Hublin, C., Kaprio, J., Partinen, M. and Koskenvuo, M. (1998) 'Sleep bruxism based on self-report in a nationwide twin cohort.' *Journal of Sleep Research, 7*(1): 61–67.

Hudson, J.L., Gradisar, M., Gamble, A., Schniering, C.A. and Rebelo, I. (2009) 'The sleep patterns and problems of clinically anxious children.' *Behaviour Research and Therapy, 47*(4): 339–344.

Hui, D.S. (2009) 'Craniofacial profile assessment in patients with obstructive sleep apnea.' *Sleep, 32*(1): 11–12. (A commentary on Lee *et al.* 'Craniofacial phenotyping in obstructive sleep apnea – a novel quantitative photographic approach.' *Sleep, 2008, 31*(1): 37–45 and Lee *et al.* 'Prediction of obstructive sleep apnea with craniofacial photographic analysis.' *Sleep, 2009, 32*: 46–52.)

Hursthouse, M.W. (1973) 'Burns from enuresis alarm apparatus: Case report.' *New Zealand Medical Journal, 79*(499): 258–259.

Huynh, N., Manzini, C., Rompré, P.H. and Lavigne, G.J. (2007) 'Weighing the potential effectiveness of various treatments for sleep bruxism.' *Journal of the Canadian Dental Association, 73*(8): 727–730.

Huynh, N.T., Rompré, P.H., Montplaisir, J.Y., Manzini, C. *et al.* (2006) 'Comparison of various treatments for sleep bruxism using determinants of number needed to treat and effect size.' *International Journal of Prosthodontics, 19*(5): 435–441.

Iglowstein, I., Jenni, O.G., Molinari, L. and Largo, R.H. (2003) 'Sleep duration from infancy to adolescence: Reference values and generational trends.' *Pediatrics, 111*(2): 302–307.

Imeri, L. and Opp, M.R. (2009) 'How (and why) the immune system makes us sleep.' *Naure Reviews: Neuroscience, 10*(3): 199–210.

Ivanenko, A. and Patwari, P.P. (2009) Recognition and Management of Pediatric Sleep Disorders.' *Primary Psychiatry, 16*(2): 42–50.

Ivanenko, A., Tauman, R. and Gozal, D. (2003) 'Modafinil in the treatment of excessive daytime sleepiness in children.' *Sleep Medicine, 4*: 579–582.

Jafferany, M. (2007) 'Psychodermatology: A guide to understanding common psychocutaneous disorders.' *Journal of Clinical Psychiatry, 9*: 203–213.

James, S.J., Melnyk, S., Fuchs, G., Reid, T. *et al.* (2009) 'Efficacy of methylcobalamin and folinic acid treatment on glutathione redox status in children with autism.' *American Journal of Clinical Nutrition, 89*(1): 425–430.

Jan, J.E. and Freeman, R.D. (2004) 'Melatonin therapy for circadian rhythm sleep disorders in children with multiple disabilities: What have we learned in the last decade?' *Developmental Medicine and Child Neurology, 46*(11): 776–782.

Jan, J.E., Freeman, R.D., Wasdell, M.B. and Bomben, M.M. (2004) 'A child with severe night terrors and sleep-walking responds to melatonin therapy.' *Developmental Medicine and Child Neurology, 46*(11): 789.

Janowitz, H.D. (2000) 'Sleep disorders in the Macbeths.' *Journal of the Royal Society of Medicine, 93*: 87–88.

Javaheri, S., Storfer-Isser, A., Rosen, C.L. and Redline, S. (2008) 'Sleep quality and elevated blood pressure in adolescents.' *Circulation, 118*(10): 1034–1040.

Jenni, O.G. and O'Connor, B.B. (2005) 'Children's sleep: An interplay between culture and biology.' *Pediatrics, 115*(1): 204–216.

Jiménez, E.G. (2011) 'Genes and obesity: A cause and effect relationship.' *Endocrinología Y Nutrición, 58*(9): 492–496.

Johns, M.W. (1991) 'A new method for measuring daytime sleepiness: The Epworth Sleepiness Scale.' *Sleep, 14*(6): 540–545.

Joly-Mascheroni, R.M., Senju, A. and Shepherd, A.J. (2008) 'Dogs catch human yawns.' *Biology Letters, 4*: 446–448.

Jones, D.P.H. and Verduyn, C.M. (1983) 'Behavioural management of sleep problems.' *Archives of Disease in Childhood, 58*: 442–444.

Jonsson, L., Ljunggren, E., Bremer, A., Pedersen, C. *et al.* (2010) 'Mutation screening of melatonin-related genes in patients with autism spectrum disorders.' BMC Medical Genomics, 3: 10. doi:10.1186/1755-9794-3-10.

Jung, H-K., Choung, R.S. and Talley, N.J. (2010) 'Gastroesophageal reflux disease and sleep disorders: Evidence for a causal link and therapeutic implications.' Journal of Neurogastroenterology and Motility, 16: 22–29.

Junien, C. (2006) 'Impact of diets and nutrients/drugs on early epigenetic programming.' Journal of Inherited Metabolic Disease, 29: 359–365.

Kaleyias, J., Cruz, M., Goraya, J.S., Valencia, I. *et al.* (2008) 'Spectrum of polysomnographic abnormalities in children with epilepsy.' Pediatric Neurology, 39(3): 170–176.

Kaplan, B., Karabay, G., Zagyapan, R.D., Ozer, C. *et al.* (2004) 'Effects of taurine in glucose and taurine administration.' *Amino Acids, 27*: 327–333.

Kato, T. and Lavigne, G.J. (2010) 'Sleep bruxism: A sleep-related movement disorder.' *Sleep Medicine Clinics, 5*: 9–35.

Kato, T., Dal-Fabbro, C. and Lavigne, G.J. (2003) 'Current knowledge on awake and sleep bruxism: Overview.' *The Alpha Omegan, 96*: 24.

Katz, E.S. and D'Ambrosio, C.M. (2010) 'Pediatric obstructive sleep apnea syndrome.' *Clinics in Chest Medicine, 31*(2): 221–234.

Kellner, R., Neidhardt, J., Krakow, B. and Pathak, D. (1991) 'Changes in chronic nightmares after one session of desensitization or rehearsal instructions.' *American Journal of Psychiatry, 149*: 659–663.

Kiddoo, D. (2007) 'Nocturnal enuresis.' *Clinical Evidence* (Online), pii:0305: 1–15.

Kimata, H. (2001) 'Effect of humor on allergen-induced wheal responses.' *Journal of the American Medical Association, 285*: 738.

Kimata, H. (2004) 'Laughter counteracts enhancement of plasma neurotrophin levels and allergic skin wheal responses by mobile phone-mediated stress.' *Behavioral Medicine, 29*: 149–152.

Kimata, H. (2007) 'Laughter elevates the levels of breast-milk melatonin.' *Journal of Psychosomatic Research, 62*(6): 699–702.

Kinney, D.K., Miller, A.M., Crowley, D.J., Huang, E. and Gerber, E. (2008a) 'Autism prevalence following prenatal exposure to hurricanes and tropical storms in Louisiana.' *Journal of Autism and Developmental Disorders, 38*: 481–488.

Kinney, D.K., Munir, K.M., Crowley, D.J. and Miller, A.M. (2008b) 'Prenatal stress and risk for autism.' *Neuroscience and Biobehavioral Reviews, 32*: 1519–1532.

Klerman, E.B., Rimmer, D.W., Dijk, D-J., Kronauer, R.E. *et al.* (1998) 'Nonphotic entrainment of the human circadian pacemaker.' *American Journal of Physiology, 274 (Regulatory Integrative and Comparative Physiology, 43)*: R991–R996.

Kohane, I.S., McMurry, A., Weber, G., MacFadden, D. *et al.* (2012) 'The co-morbidity burden of children and young adults with autism spectrum disorders.' PLoS ONE, 7(4): e33224. doi:10.1371/journal.pone.0033224.

Kothare, S.V. and Kaleyias, J. (2008) 'Narcolepsy and other hypersomnias in children.' *Current Opinion in Pediatrics, 20*(6): 666–675.

Krakow, B., Lowry, C., Germain, A., Gaddy, L. *et al.* (2000) 'A retrospective study on improvements in nightmares and post-traumatic stress disorder following treatment for co-morbid sleep-disordered breathing.' *Journal of Psychosomatic Research, 49*: 291–298.

Krakow, B., Sandoval, D., Schrader, R., Keuhne, B. *et al.* (2001) 'Treatment of chronic nightmares in adjudicated adolescent girls in a residential facility.' *Journal of Adolescent Health, 29*: 94–100.

Krakowiak, P., Walker, C.K., Bremer, A.A., Baker, A.S. *et al.* (2012) 'Maternal metabolic conditions and risk for autism and other neurodevelopmental disorders.' *Pediatrics, 129*(5): 1–8.

Krueger, J.M. (2008) 'The role of cytokines in sleep regulation.' *Current Pharmaceutical Design, 14*(32): 3408–3416.

Kruskal, B. (2009) 'It couldn't hurt… Could it?' Safety of complementary and alternative medicine practices.' *Acta Paediatrica, 98*: 628–630.

Krueger, J.M., Obal Jr, F. and Fang, J. (1999) 'Why we sleep: A theoretical view of sleep function.' *Sleep Medicine Reviews, 3*(2): 119–129.

Kryger, M.H., Otake, K. and Foerster, J. (2002) 'Low body stores of iron and restless legs syndrome: A correctable cause of insomnia in adolescents and teenagers.' *Sleep Medicine, 3*(2): 127–132.

Kryger, M.H., Walld, R. and Manfreda, J. (2002) 'Diagnoses received by narcolepsy patients in the year prior to diagnosis by a sleep specialist.' *Sleep, 25*(1): 36–41.

Laakso, M.L., Lindblom, N., Leinonen, L. and Kaski, M. (2007) 'Endogenous melatonin predicts efficacy of exogenous melatonin in consolidation of fragmented wrist-activity rhythm of adult patients with developmental brain disorders: A double-blind, placebo-controlled, crossover study.' *Sleep Medicine, 8*(3): 222–239.

Laberge, L., Petit, D., Simard, C., Vitaro, F., Tremblay, R.E. and Montplaisir, J. (2001) 'Development of sleep patterns in early adolescence.' *Journal of Sleep Research, 10*: 59–67.

Lamerz, A,. Kuepper-Nybelen, J., Bruning, N., Wehle, C. *et al.* (2005) 'Prevalence of obesity, binge eating, and night eating in a cross-sectional field survey of 6-year-old children and their parents in a German urban population.' *Journal of Child Psychology and Psychiatry, 46*: 385–393.

Lancee, J., Spoormaker, V.I., Krakow, B. and van den Bout, J. (2008) 'A systematic review of cognitive-behavioral treatment for nightmares: Toward a well-established treatment.' *Journal of Clinical Sleep Medicine, 4*(5): 475–480.

Lancee, J., Spoormaker, V.I., Peterse, G. and van den Bout, J. (2008) 'Measuring nightmare frequency: Retrospective questionnaires versus prospective logs.' *Open Sleep Journal*, 1: 26–28.

Lang, R., White, P.J., Machalicek, W., Rispoli, M. *et al.* (2009) 'Treatment of bruxism in individuals with developmental disabilities: A systematic review.' *Research in Developmental Disabilities, 30*(5): 809–818.

Lask, B. (1988) 'Novel and non-toxic treatment for night terrors.' *British Medical Journal, 297*: 592.

Lavie, P., Pillar, G. and Malhotra, A. (2005) 'Further Reading.' In: *Sleep Disorders: Diagnosis, Management and Treatment. A Handbook for Clinicians.* London: Martin Dunitz.

Lavigne, G.J. and Montplaisir, J.Y. (1994) 'Restless legs syndrome and sleep bruxism: Prevalence and association among Canadians.' Sleep, 17: 739–743.

Leboeuf, C., Brown, P., Herman, A., Leembruggen, K. *et al.* (1991) 'Chiropractic care of children with nocturnal enuresis: A prospective outcome study.' Journal of Manipulative & Physiological Therapeutics, 14(2): 110–115.

LeBourgeois, M.K., Giannotti, F., Cortesi, F., Wolfson, A. and Harsh, J. (2004) 'Sleep hygiene and sleep quality in Italian and American adolescents.' Annals of the New York Academy of Science, 1021: 352–354.

LeBourgeois, M.K., Giannotti, F., Cortesi, F., Wolfson, A.R. and Harsh, J. (2005) 'The relationship between reported sleep quality and sleep hygiene in Italian and American adolescents.' Pediatrics, 115: 257–265.

Lei, D., Ma, J., Shen, X., Du, X. *et al.* (2012) 'Changes in the brain microstructure of children with primary monosymptomatic nocturnal enuresis: A diffusion tensor imaging study.' PLoS ONE, 7(2): e31023. doi:10.1371/journal.pone.0031023.

Leu, R.M., Beyderman, L., Botzolakis, E.J., Surdyka, K. *et al.* (2010) 'Relation of melatonin to sleep architecture in children with autism.' Journal of Autism and Developmental Disorders, Online First. doi: 10.1007/s10803-010-1072-1.

Lewandowski, A.S., Toliver-Sokol, M. and Palermo, T.M. (2011) 'Evidence-based review of subjective pediatric sleep measures.' Journal of Pediatric Psychology, 58(3): 699–713.

Licis, A.K., Desruisseau, D.M., Yamada, K.A., Duntley, S.P. and Gurnett, C.A. (2011) 'Novel genetic findings in an extended family pedigree with sleepwalking.' Neurology, 76: 49–52.

Lim, A., Cranswick, N. and South, M. (2010) 'Adverse events associated with the use of complementary and alternative medicine in children.' Archives of Disease in Childhood, 96(3): 297–300. doi:10.1136/2 of 4 adc.2010.183152.

Limoges, E., Mottron, L., Bolduc, C., Berthiaume, C. and Godbout, R. (2005) 'Atypical sleep architecture and the autism phenotype.' Brain, 128: 1049–1061.

Limperopoulos, C., Bassan, H., Sullivan, N.R., Soul, J.S. *et al.* (2008) 'Positive screening for autism in ex-preterm infants: Prevalence and risk factors.' Pediatrics, 121: 758–765.

Lipton, A.J. and Gozal, D. (2003) 'Treatment of obstructive sleep apnea in children: Do we really know how?' Sleep Medicine Reviews, 7: 61–80.

Littner, M., Johnson, S.F., McCall, W.V., Anderson, W.M. *et al.* (2001) 'Practice parameters for the treatment of narcolepsy: An update for 2000.' Sleep, 24: 451–466.

Liukkonen, K., Virkkula, P., Aronen, E.T., Kirjavainen, T. and Pitkaranta, A. (2008) 'All snoring is not adenoids in young children.' International Journal of Pediatric Otorhinolaryngology, 72: 879–884.

Lombroso, C.T. (2000) 'Pavor nocturnus of proven epileptic origin.' Epilepsia, 41(9): 1221–1226.

Lopez-Wagner, M.C., Hoffman, C.D., Sweeney, D.P., Hodge, D. and Gilliam, J.E. (2008) 'Sleep problems of parents of typically developing children and parents of children with autism.' *Journal of Genetic Psychology, 169*(3): 245–259.

Lorimer, P.A., Simpson, R.L., Myles, B.S. and Ganz, J.B. (2002) 'The use of social stories as a preventative behavioral intervention in a home setting with a child with autism.' *Journal of Positive Behavioral Intervention, 4*(1): 53–60.

Lozoff, B. and Georgieff, M.K. (2006) 'Iron deficiency and brain development.' *Seminars in Pediatric Neurology, 13*: 158–165.

Lukusa, T., Vermeesch, J.R., Holvoet, M., Fryns, J.P. and Devriendt, K. (2004) 'Deletion 2q37.3 and autism: Molecular cytogenetic mapping of the candidate region for autistic disorder.' *Genetic Counselling, 15*(3): 293–301.

Lumeng, J.C. and Chervin, R.D. (2008) 'Epidemiology of pediatric obstructive sleep apnea.' *Proceedings of the American Thoracic Society, 5*: 242–252.

Lundgren, J., Allison, K. and Stunkard, A. (2006) 'Familial aggregation in the night eating syndrome.' *International Journal of Eating Disorders, 39*(6): 516–518.

Lyon, C. and Schnall, J. (2010) 'What is the best treatment for nocturnal enuresis in children?' *Journal of Family Practice, 54*(10): 905–909.

McArthur A.J. and Budden, S.S. (1998) 'Sleep dysfunction in Rett syndrome: A trial of exogenous melatonin treatment.' *Developmental Medicine and Child Neurology, 40*(3): 186–192.

McDermott, S., Zhou, L. and Mann, J. (2008) 'Injury treatment among children with autism or pervasive developmental disorder.' *Journal of Autism and Developmental Disorders, 38*(4): 626–633.

McGowan, P.O., Meaney, M.J. and Szyf, M. (2008) 'Diet and the epigenetic (re) programming of phenotypic differences in behavior.' *Brain Research, 1237*: 12–24.

McKenna, J.J. and McDade, T. (2005) 'Why babies should never sleep alone: A review of the co-sleeping controversy in relation to SIDS, bedsharing and breast feeding.' *Paediatric Respiratory Reviews, 6*: 134–152.

McKenna, J.J., Thoman, E., Anders T.E., Sadeh, A. *et al.* (1993) 'Infant–parent co-sleeping in evolutionary perspective: Implications for understanding infant sleep development and the sudden infant death syndrome (SIDS).' *Sleep, 16*: 263–282.

Machado-Vieira, R., Viale, C.I. and Kapczinski, F. (2001) 'Mania associated with an energy drink: The possible role of caffeine, taurine, and inositol.' *Canadian Journal of Psychiatry, 46*(5): 454–455.

Makley, M.J., English, J.B., Drubach, D.A., Kreuz, A.J. *et al.* (2008) 'Prevalence of sleep disturbance in closed head injury patients in a rehabilitation unit.' *Neurorehabilitation and Neural Repair, 22*(4): 341–347.

Malow, B.A., McGrew, S.G., Harvey, M., Henderson, L.M. and Stone, W.L. (2006) 'Impact of treating sleep apnea in a child with autism spectrum disorder.' *Pediatric Neurology, 34*: 325–328.

Mamelak, M., Black, J., Montplaisir, J. and Ristanovic, R. (2004) 'A pilot study on the effects of sodium oxybate on sleep architecture and daytime alertness in narcolepsy.' *Sleep, 27*(7): 1327–1334.

Manfredini, D. and Lobbenzoo, F. (2009) 'Role of psychosocial factors in the etiology of bruxism.' *Journal of Orofacial Pain, 23*(2): 153–166.

Manni, R. and Terzaghi, M. (2010) 'Comorbidity between epilepsy and sleep disorders.' *Epilepsy Research, 90*: 171–177.

Marks, I.M. (1978) 'Rehearsal relief of a nightmare.' *British Journal of Psychiatry, 135*: 461–465.

Marshall, J. and Meltzoff, A.N. (2011) 'Neural mirroring systems: Exploring the EEG mu rhythm in human infancy.' *Developmental Cognitive Neuroscience, 1*(2): 110–123.

Martínez-Rodríguez, J.E., Lin, L., Iranzo, A., Genis, D. *et al.* (2003) 'Decreased hypocretin-1 (orexin-A) levels in the cerebrospinal fluid of patients with myotonic dystrophy and excessive daytime sleepiness.' *Sleep, 26*(3): 287–290.

Martynska, L., Wolinska-Witort, E., Chmielowska, M., Bik, W. and Baranowska, B. (2005) 'The physiological role of orexins.' *Neuroendocrinology Letters, 2*(4): 289–292.

Matos, G., Andersen, M.L., do Valle, A.C. and Tufik, S. (2010) 'The relationship between sleep and epilepsy: Evidence from clinical trials and animal models.' *Journal of the Neurological Sciences, 295*(1): 1–7.

Mayer, G., Wilde-Frenz, J. and Kurella, B. (2007) 'Sleep related rhythmic movement disorder revisited.' *Journal of Sleep Research, 16*: 110–116.

Mayes, S.D., Calhoun, S.L., Bixler, E.O., Vgontzas, A.N. *et al.* (2009) 'ADHD subtypes and comorbid anxiety, depression, and oppositional-defiant disorder: Differences in sleep problems.' *Journal of Pediatric Psychology, 34*(3): 328–337.

Mehra, R. and Redline, S. (2008) 'Sleep apnea: A proinflammatory disorder that coaggregates with obesity.' *Journal of Allergy and Clinical Immunology, 121*(5): 1096–1102.

Melke, J., Goubran-Botros, H., Chaste, P., Betancur, C. *et al.* (2008) 'Abnormal melatonin synthesis in autism spectrum disorders.' *Molecular Psychiatry, 13*(1): 90–98.

Mennella, J.A. and Garcia-Gomez, P.L. (2001) 'Sleep disturbances after acute exposure to alcohol in mothers' milk.' *Alcohol, 25*(3): 153–158.

Merlino, G., Serafini, A., Robiony, F., Valente, M. and Gigli, G.L. (2009) 'Restless legs syndrome: Differential diagnosis and management with rotigotine.' *Neuropsychiatric Disease and Treatment, 5*: 67–80.

Miano, S. and Ferri, R. (2010) 'Epidemiology and management of insomnia in children with autistic spectrum disorders.' *Paediatric Drugs, 12*(2): 75–84.

Miano, S., Bruni, O., Elia, M., Trovato, A. *et al.* (2007) 'Sleep in children with autistic spectrum disorder: A questionnaire and polysomnographic study.' *Sleep Medicine, 9*(1): 64–70.

Miano, S., Paolino, M.C., Peraita-Adrados, R., Montesano, M. *et al.* (2009) 'Prevalence of EEG paroxysmal activity in a population of children with obstructive sleep apnea syndrome.' *Sleep, 32*(4): 522–529.

Mignot, E. (1998) 'Genetic and familial aspects of narcolepsy.' *Neurology, 50(Suppl 1)*: S16–S22.

Mignot, E. (2008) 'Excessive daytime sleepiness: Population and etiology versus nosology.' *Sleep Medicine Reviews, 12*: 87–94.

Mignot, E., Taheri, S. and Nishino, S. (2002) 'Sleeping with the hypothalamus: Emerging therapeutic targets for sleep disorders.' *Nature Neuroscience Supplement, 5*: 1071–1075.

Mignot, E., van Lammers, G., Ripley, B., Okun, M. *et al.* (2002) 'The role of cerebrospinal fluid hypocretin measurement in the diagnosis of narcolepsy and other hypersomnias.' *Archives of Neurology, 59*(10): 1553–1562.

Miller, K.E. (2008) 'Energy drinks, race, and problem behaviors among college students.' *Journal of Adolescent Health, 43*(5): 490–497.

Miller, W.R. and DiPilato, M. (1983) 'Treatment of nightmares via relaxation and desensitisation: A controlled evaluation.' *Journal of Consulting Clinical Psychology, 51*: 870–877.

Mindell, J.A. (1999) 'Empirically supported treatments in pediatric psychology: Bedtime refusal and night wakings in young children.' *Journal of Pediatric Psychology, 24*(6): 465–481.

Mindell, J.A., Meltzer, L.J., Carskadon, M.A. and Chervin, R.D. (2009) 'Developmental aspects of sleep hygiene: Findings from the 2004 National Sleep Foundation Sleep in America Poll.' *Sleep Medicine, 10*: 771–779.

Montgomery, P. and Dunne, D. (2007) 'Sleep disorders in children.' Clinical Evidence (Online), 2007, 09: 2304.

Moon, E.C., Corkum, P. and Smith, I.M. (2010) 'Case study: A case-series evaluation of a behavioral sleep intervention for three children with autism and primary insomnia.' *Journal of Pediatric Psychology, 36*(1): 47–54. doi:10.1093/jpepsy/jsq057.

Moore, M., Meltzer, L.J. and Mindell, J.A. (2008) 'Bedtime problems and night wakings in children.' *Primary Care, 35*(3): 569–581.

Moore, P.S. (2004) 'The use of social stories in a psychology service for children with learning disabilities: A case study of a sleep problem.' *British Journal of Learning Disabilities, 32*(3): 133–138.

Morgenthaler, T.I., Kapur, V.K., Brown, T., Swick, T.J. *et al.* (2007) 'Standards of Practice Committee of the American Academy of Sleep Medicine. Practice parameters for the treatment of narcolepsy and other hypersomnias of central origin.' *Sleep, 30*(12): 1705–1711.

Morton, J. (2004) *Understanding Developmental Disorders: A Causal Modelling Approach.* Oxford: Blackwell.

Mowrer, O.H. and Mowrer, W.M. (1938) 'Enuresis: A method for its study and treatment.' *American Journal of Orthopsychiatry, 8*: 436–459.

Mukaddes, N.M., Kilincaslan, A., Kucukyazici, G., Sevketoglu, T. and Tuncer, S. (2007) 'Autism in visually impaired individuals.' *Psychiatry and Clinical Neurosciences, 61*(1): 39–44.

Mulvaney, S.A., Kaemingk, K.L., Goodwin, J.L. and Quan, S.F. (2006) 'Parent-rated behavior problems associated with overweight before and after controlling for sleep disordered breathing.' *BMC Pediatrics, 6*: 34. doi:10.1186/1471-2431-6-34.

Muris, P., Merckelbach, H., Gadet, B. and Moulaert, V. (2000) 'Fears, worries, and scary dreams in 4- to 12-year-old children: Their content, developmental pattern, and origins.' *Journal of Clinical Child Psychology, 29*: 43–52.

Murphy, B.F. (1974) 'Hazards of children's vitamin preparations containing iron.' *Journal of the American Medical Association, 229*(3): 324.

Murray, L. and Cooper, P. (1997) 'The impact of postpartum depression on child development.' *International Review of Psychiatry, 8*(1): 55–63.

Muthu, M.S. and Prathibha, K.M. (2008) 'Management of a child with autism and severe bruxism: A case report.' *Journal of the Indian Society of Pedodontics and Preventive Dentistry, 26*(2): 82–84.

Nader, N., Chrousos, G.P. and Kino, T. (2010) 'Interactions of the circadian clock system and the HPA axis.' *Trends in Endocrinology and Metabolism, 21*(5): 277–286.

Nappo, S., Del Gado, R., Chiozza, M.L., Biraghi, M., Ferrara, P. and Caione, P. (2002) 'Nocturnal enuresis in the adolescent: A neglected problem.' *BJU International, 90*: 912–917.

Nevéus, T., Cnattingius, S., Olsson, U. and Hetta, J. (2001) 'Sleep habits and sleep problems among a community sample of schoolchildren.' *Acta Paediatrica, 90*(12): 1450–1455.

Newell, K.M., Incledon, T., Bodfish, J.W. and Sprague, R.L. (1999) 'Variability of stereotypic body-rocking in adults with mental retardation.' *American Journal of Mental Retardation, 104*: 279–288.

Nguyen, B.H., Pérusse, D., Paquet, J., Petit, D. *et al.* (2008) 'Sleep terrors in children: A prospective study of twins.' *Pediatrics, 122*(6): e1164–1167.

Nicholas, B., Rudrasingham, V., Nash, S., Kirov, G., Owen, M.J. and Wimpory, D.C. (2007) 'Association of Per1 and Npas2 with autistic disorder: Support for the clock genes/social timing hypothesis.' *Molecular Psychiatry, 12*: 581–592.

Nielsen, T.A., Stenstrom, P. and Levin, R. (2006) 'Nightmare frequency as a function of age, gender, and September 11, 2001: Findings from an internet questionnaire.' *Dreaming, 16*(3): 145–158.

Nieto, F.J., Peppard, P.E. and Young, T.B. (2009) 'Sleep disordered breathing and metabolic syndrome.' *Western Medical Journal, 108*(5): 263–265.

Nishida, M., Pearsall, J., Buckner, R.L. and Walker, M.P. (2009) 'REM sleep, prefrontal theta, and the consolidation of human emotional memory.' *Cerebral Cortex, 19*: 1158–1166.

Nishino, S. and Mignot, E. (1997) 'Pharmacological Aspects of Human and Canine Narcolepsy.' *Progress in Neurobiology, 52*(1): 27–78.

Nobili, L., Francione, S., Mai, R., Cardinale, F. *et al.* (2007) 'Surgical treatment of drug-resistant nocturnal frontal lobe epilepsy.' *Brain, 130*(2): 561–573.

Nguyen, A.T., Rauch, T.A., Pfeifer, G.P. and Hu, V.W. (2010) 'Global methylation profiling of lymphoblastoid cell lines reveals epigenetic contributions to autism spectrum disorders and a novel autism candidate gene, RORA, whose protein product is reduced in autistic brain.' *FASEB Journal, 24*(8): 3036–3051.

Obermann, M., Schorn, C.F., Mummel, P., Kastrup, O. and Maschke, M. (2006) 'Taurine induced toxic encephalopathy?' *Clinical Neurology and Neurosurgery, 108*: 812–813.

O'Brien, L.M., Holbrook, C.R., Mervis, C.B., Klaus, C.J. *et al.* (2003a) 'Sleep and neurobehavioral characteristics of 5- to 7-year-old children with parentally reported symptoms of attention-deficit/hyperactivity disorder.' *Pediatrics, 111*(3): 554–563.

O'Brien, L.M., Ivanenko, A., Crabtree, V.M., Holbrook, C.R. *et al.* (2003b) 'The effect of stimulants on sleep characteristics in children with attention deficit/hyperactivity disorder.' *Sleep Medicine, 4*(4): 309–316.

O'Callaghan, F.J., Clarke, A.A., Hancock, E., Hunt, A. and Osborne J.P. (1999) 'Use of melatonin to treat sleep disorders in tuberous sclerosis.' *Developmental Medicine and Child Neurology, 41*: 123–126.

O'Connor , M-F., Bower, J.E., Cho, H.J., Creswell, J.D. *et al.* (2009) 'To assess, to control, to exclude: Effects of biobehavioral factors on circulating inflammatory markers.' *Brain, Behavior, and Immunity, 23*: 887–897.

O'Connor, T.G., Caprariello, P., Blackmore, E.R., Gregory, A.M. *et al.* (2007) 'Prenatal mood disturbance predicts sleep problems in infancy and toddlerhood.' *Early Human Development, 83*(7): 451–458.

Oguni, H. (2011) 'Treatment of benign focal epilepsies in children: When and how should they be treated?' Brain and Development, 33(3): 2017–212.

Ohayon, M.M. (2008) 'From wakefulness to excessive sleepiness: What we know and still need to know.' *Sleep Medicine Reviews, 12*: 129–141.

Ohayon, M.M., Guilleminault, C. and Priest R.G. (1999) 'Night terrors, sleepwalking, and confusional arousals in the general population: Their frequency and relationship to other sleep and mental disorders.' *Journal of Clinical Psychiatry, 60*(4): 268–276.

Ommerborn, M.A., Schneider, C., Giraki, M., Schafer, R. *et al.* (2007) 'Effects of an occlusal splint compared with cognitive-behavioral treatment on sleep bruxism activity.' *European Journal of Oral Science, 115*(1): 7–14.

Orbach, D., Ritaccio, A. and Devinsky, O. (2003) 'Psychogenic, nonepileptic seizures associated with video-EEG-verified sleep.' *Epilepsia, 44*(1): 64–68.

O'Reardon, J.P., Stunkard, A.J. and Allison, K.C. (2004) 'Clinical trial of sertraline in the treatment of night eating syndrome.' *International Journal of Eating Disorders, 35*(1): 16–26.

O'Reilly, M.F. (1995) 'Functional analysis and treatment of escape-maintained aggression correlated with sleep deprivation.' *Journal of Applied Behaviour Analysis, 28*: 225–226.

Orr, W.C., Robert, J.J.T., Houck, J.R., Giddens, C.L. and Tawk, M.M. (2009) 'The effect of acid suppression on upper airway anatomy and obstruction in patients with sleep apnea and gastroesophageal reflux disease.' *Journal of Clinical Sleep Medicine, 5*(4): 330–334.

Oudiette, D., Constantinescu, I., Leclair-Visonneau, L., Vidailhet, M. *et al.* (2011) 'Evidence for the re-enactment of a recently learned behavior during sleepwalking.' *PLoS ONE, 6*(3): e18056. doi:10.1371/journal.pone.0018056.

Owens, J.A. (2005) 'The ADHD and sleep conundrum: A review.' *Developmental and Behavioral Pediatrics, 26*(4): 312–322.

Owens, J.A. and Dalzell, V. (2005) 'Use of the "BEARS" sleep screening tool in a pediatric residents' continuity clinic: A pilot study.' *Sleep Medicine, 6*: 63–69.

Owens, J.A., Opipari, L., Nobile, C. and Spirito, A. (1998) 'Sleep and daytime behavior in children with obstructive sleep apnea and behavioral sleep disorders.' *Pediatrics, 102*(5): 1178–1184.

Owens, J.A., Spirito, A. and McGuinn, M. (2000) 'The Children's Sleep Habits Questionnaire (CSHQ): Psychometric properties of a survey instrument for school-aged children.' *Sleep, 23*: 1043–1051.

Owens, J.A., Spirito, A., McGuinn, M. and Nobile, C. (2000) 'Sleep habits and sleep disturbance in elementary school-aged children.' *Journal of Developmental and Behavioral Pediatrics, 21*: 27–36.

Palace, E.M. and Johnston, C. (1989) 'Treatment of recurrent nightmares by the dream reorganization approach.' *Journal of Behavior Therapy and Experimental Psychiatry, 20*(3): 219–226.

Palagini, L. and Rosenlicht, N. (2010) 'Sleep, dreaming, and mental health: A review of historical and neurobiological perspectives.' *Sleep Medicine Reviews, 15*(3):179–186. doi:10.1016/j.smrv.2010.07.003.

Pallesen, S., Nordhus, I.H., Nielsen, G.H., Havik, O.E. *et al.* (2001) 'Prevalence of insomnia in the adult Norwegian population.' *Sleep, 24*(7): 771–779.

Palombini, L., Pelayo, R. and Guilleminault, C. (2004) 'Efficacy of automated continuous positive airway pressure in children with sleep-related breathing disorders in an attended setting.' *Pediatrics, 113*: e412–e417.

Panayiotopoulos, C.P., Michael, M., Sanders, S., Valeta, T. and Koutroumanidis, M. (2008) 'Benign childhood focal epilepsies: Assessment of established and newly recognized syndromes. *Brain, 131*: 2264–2286.

Paparrigopoulos, T.J. (2005) 'REM sleep behaviour disorder: Clinical profiles and pathophysiology.' *International Review of Psychiatry, 17*(4): 293–300.

Patel, A., Schieble, T., Davidson, C., Tran, M.C.J. *et al.* (2006) 'Distraction with a hand-held video game reduces pediatric preoperative anxiety.' *Pediatric Anaesthesia, 16*: 1019–1027.

Patel, S.R., Malhotra, A., White, D.P., Gottlieb, D.J. and Hu, F.B. (2006) 'Association between reduced sleep and weight gain in women.' *American Journal of Epidemiology, 164*: 947–954.

Paterson, G.R. (1982) *A Social Learning Approach 3: Coercive Family Process.* Eugene, OR: Castalia Press.

Pelc, K., Cheron, G., Boyd, S.G. and Dan, B. (2008) 'Are there distinctive sleep problems in Angelman syndrome?' *Sleep Medicine,* 9(4): 434–441.

Perry, A., Bentin, S., Shalev, I., Israel, S. *et al.* (2010) 'Intranasal oxytocin modulates EEG mu/alpha and beta rhythms during perception of biological motion.' *Psychoneuroendocrinology,* 35(10): 1446–1453. doi:10.1016/j.psyneuen.2010.04.011.

Peters, J.M., Camfield, C.S. and Camfield, P.R. (2001) 'Population study of benign rolandic epilepsy: Is treatment needed?' *Neurology,* 57(3): 537–539.

Peterson, J.L. and Peterson, M. (2003) *The Sleep Fairy.* Omaha, NE: Behave'n Kids Press.

Peyron, C., Faraco, J., Rogers, W., Ripley, B. *et al.* (2000) 'A mutation in a case of early onset narcolepsy and a generalized absence of hypocretin peptides in human narcoleptic brains.' *Nature Medicine,* 6(9): 991–997.

Phillips, D.A., Watson, A.R. and MacKinlay, D. (1998) 'Distress and the micturating cystourethrogram: Does preparation help?' *Acta Paediatrica,* 87(2): 175–179.

Piazza, C.C. and Fisher, W. (1991) 'A faded bedtime with response cost protocol for treatment of multiple sleep problems in children.' *Journal of Applied Behaviour Analysis,* 24: 129–140.

Piazza, C.C., Fisher, W. and Sherer, M. (1997) 'Treatment of multiple sleep problems in children with developmental disabilities: Faded bedtime with response cost versus bedtime scheduling.' *Developmental Medicine and Child Neurology,* 39(6): 414–418.

Picchietti, D.L. and Stevens, H.E. (2008) 'Early manifestations of restless legs syndrome in childhood and adolescence.' *Sleep Medicine,* 9: 770–781.

Picchietti, D.L., Rajendran, R.R., Wilson, M.P. and Picchietti, M.A. (2009) 'Pediatric restless legs syndrome and periodic limb movement disorder: Parent–child pairs.' *Sleep Medicine,* 10: 925–931.

Picchietti, M.A. and Picchietti, D.L. (2008) 'Restless legs syndrome and periodic limb movement disorder in children and adolescents.' *Seminars in Pediatric Neurology,* 15: 91–99.

Pierce, C.J. and Gale, E.N. (1988) 'A comparison of different treatments for nocturnal bruxism.' *Journal of Dental Research,* 67(3): 597–601.

Pierce, K. (2011) 'Early functional brain development in autism and the promise of sleep fMRI.' *Brain Research,* 1380: 162–174.

Pigeon, W.R. and Yurcheshen, M. (2009) 'Behavioral sleep medicine interventions for restless legs syndrome and periodic limb movement disorder.' *Sleep Medicine Clinics,* 4: 487–494.

Platek, S.M., Critton, S.R., Myers, T.E. and Gallup Jr, G.G. (2003) 'Contagious yawning: The role of self-awareness and mental state attribution.' *Cognitive Brain Research,* 17: 223–227.

Ponde, M.P., Novaes, C.N. and Losapio, M.F. (2010) 'Frequency of symptoms of attention deficit and hyperactivity disorder in autistic children.' *Arquivos de Neuro-psiquiatria,* 68(1): 103–106.

Popoviciu, L. and Corfariu, O. (1983) 'Efficacy and safety of midazolam in the treatment of night terrors in children.' *British Journal of Clinical Pharmacology,* 16: 97S–102S.

Provine, R.R. (1989) 'Faces as releasers of contagious yawning: An approach to face detection using normal human subjects, *Bulletin of the Psychonomic Society,* 27: 211–214.

Ramoz, N., Cai, G., Reichert, J.G., Corwin, T.E. *et al.* (2006) 'Family-based association study of TPH1 and TPH2 polymorphisms in autism.' *American Journal of Medical Genetics B: Neuropsychiatric Genetics,* 141B(8): 861–867.

Randazzo, A.C., Muehlbach, M.J., Schweitzer, P.K. and Walsh, J.K. (1988) 'Cognitive function following acute sleep restriction in children ages 10–14.' *Sleep, 21*(8): 861–868.

Rantala, H. and Putkonen, T. (1999) 'Occurrence, outcome and prognostic factors of infantile spasms and Lennox-Gastaut syndrome.' *Epilepsia, 40*: 286–289.

Rao, V., Spiro, J., Vaishnavi, S., Rastogi, P. *et al.* (2008) 'Prevalence and types of sleep disturbances acutely after traumatic brain injury.' *Brain Injury, 22*(5): 381–386.

Rechtschaffen, I.A. (1971) 'The control of sleep.' In: W.A. Hunt (ed.) *Human Behavior and Its Control.* Cambridge, MA: Shenkman Publishing Co.

Redcay, E. and Courchesne, E. (2008) 'Deviant functional magnetic resonance imaging patterns of brain activity to speech in 2–3-year-old children with autism spectrum disorder.' *Biological Psychiatry, 64*: 589–598.

Redline, S., Storfer-Isser, A., Rosen, C.L., Johnson, N.L. *et al.* (2007) 'Association between metabolic syndrome and sleep-disordered breathing in adolescents.' *American Journal of Respiratory and Critical Care Medicine, 176*: 401–408.

Reed, W.R., Beavers, S., Reddy, S.K. and Kern, G. (1994) 'Chiropractic management of primary nocturnal enuresis.' *Journal of Manipulative & Physiological Therapeutics, 17*(9): 596–600.

Reghunandanan, V. and Reghunandanan, R. (2006) 'Neurotransmitters of the suprachiasmatic nuclei.' *Journal of Circadian Rhythms, 4*: 2. doi:10.1186/1740-3391-4-2.

Reid, M.J., Walter, A.L. and O'Leary, S.G. (1999) 'Treatment of young children's bedtime refusal and nighttime wakings: A comparison of "standard" and graduated ignoring procedures.' *Journal of Abnormal Child Psychology, 27*(1): 5–16.

Reilly, J.J., Armstrong, J., Dorosty, A.R., Emmett, P.M. *et al.* (2005) 'Early life risk factors for obesity in childhood: Cohort study.' *British Medical Journal, 330*: 1357.

Revonsuo, A. (2000) 'The reinterpretation of dreams: An evolutionary hypothesis of the function of dreaming.' Behavioral and Brain Sciences, 23: 877–901.

Revonsuo, A. and Valli, K. (2008) 'How to test the threat simulation theory.' *Consciousness and Cognition, 17*: 1292–1296.

Rial, R.V., Nicolau, M.C., Gamundi, A., Akaarir, M. *et al.* (2007) 'The trivial function of sleep.' *Sleep Medicine Reviews, 11*: 311–325.

Richdale, A.L. and Prior, M.R. (1992) 'Urinary cortisol circadian rhythm in a group of high-functioning autistic children.' *Journal of Autism and Developmental Disorders, 22*(3): 443–447.

Richardson, H.L., Walker, A.M. and Horne, R.S.C. (2009) 'Maternal smoking impairs arousal patterns in sleeping infants.' *Sleep, 32*(4): 515–521.

Rickert, V.I. and Johnson, C.M. (1988) 'Reducing nocturnal awakening and crying episodes in infants and young children: A comparison between scheduled awakenings and systematic ignoring.' *Pediatrics, 81*(2): 203–212.

Riemann, D. and Perlis, M.L. (2009) 'The treatments of chronic insomnia: A review of benzodiazepine receptor agonists and psychological and behavioral therapies.' *Sleep Medicine Reviews, 13*(3): 205–214.

Rodwin, M.A. (2011) *Conflicts of Interest and the Future of Medicine: The United States, France, and Japan.* Oxford: Oxford University Press.

Rohdin, M., Fernell, E., Eriksson, M., Albåge, M., Lagercrantz, H. and Katz-Salamon, M. (2007) 'Disturbances in cardiorespiratory function during day and night in Rett syndrome.' *Pediatric Neurology, 37*(5): 338–344.

Romcy-Pereira, R.N., Leite, J.P. and Garcia-Cairasco, N. (2009) 'Synaptic plasticity along the sleep–wake cycle: Implications for epilepsy.' *Epilepsy & Behavior, 14*: 47–53.

Rosenwasser, A.M. (2009) 'Functional neuroanatomy of sleep and circadian rhythms.' *Brain Research Reviews, 61*: 281–306.

Roth, T. (2007) 'Insomnia: definition, prevalence, etiology, and consequences.' *Journal of Clinical Sleep Medicine, 3*(Suppl 5): S7–S10.

Sack, U., Burkhardt, U., Borte, M., Schadlich, H. *et al.* (1998) 'Age-dependent levels of select immunological mediators in sera of healthy children.' *Clinical and Diagnostic Laboratory Immunology, 5*(1): 28–32.

Sadeghi, M., Daniel, V., Naujokat, C., Weimer, R. and Opelz, G. (2005) 'Strikingly higher interleukin (IL)1a , IL-1b and soluble interleukin-1 receptor antagonist (sIL-1RA) but similar IL-2, sIL-2R, IL-3, IL-4, IL-6, sIL-6R, IL-10, tumour necrosis factor (TNF)-a, transforming growth factor (TGF)-b 2 and interferon IFN-g urine levels in healthy females compared to healthy males: protection against urinary tract injury?' *Clinical and Experimental Immunology, 142*(2): 312–317.

Sadeh, A. (2004). 'A brief screening questionnaire for infant sleep problems: Validation and findings for an internet sample.' *Pediatrics, 113*(6): 570–577.

Sadeh, A., Raviv, A. and Gruber, R. (2000) 'Sleep patterns and sleep disruptions in school-age children.' *Developmental Psychology, 36*: 291–301.

Sadeh, A. and Sivan, Y. (2009) 'Clinical practice: Sleep problems during infancy.' *European Journal of Pediatrics, 168*(10): 1159–1164.

Sajith, S.G. and Clarke, D. (2007) 'Melatonin and sleep disorders associated with intellectual disability: A clinical review.' *Journal of Intellectual Disability Research, 51*(1): 2–13.

Salzarulo, P. and Chevalier, A. (1983) 'Sleep problems in children and their relationship with early disturbances of the waking-sleeping rhythms.' *Sleep, 6*: 47–51.

Sangal, B., Owens, J., Allen, A., Sutton, V. *et al.* (2006) 'Effects of atomoxetine and methylphenidate on children with attention deficit hyperactivity disorder.' *Sleep, 29*(12): 1573–1585.

Scharf, M.T., Naidoo, N., Zimmerman, J.E. and Pack, A.I. (2008) 'The energy hypothesis of sleep revisited.' *Progress in Neurobiology, 86*: 264–280.

Schenck, C.H. and Mahowald, M.W. (2006) 'Topiramate therapy of sleep related eating disorder (SRED).' *Sleep, 29*: A268.

Schenck, C.H., Connoy, D.A., Castellanos, M., Johnson, B. *et al.* (2005) 'Zolpidem-induced sleep-related eating disorder (SRED) in 19 patients.' *Sleep, 28*: A259.

Schmoll, C., Lascaratos, G., Dhillon, B., Skene, D. *et al.* (2010) 'The role of retinal regulation of sleep in health and disease.' *Sleep Medicine Reviews, 15*(2): 107–113.

Schnetz-Boutaud, N.C., Anderson, B.M., Brown, K.D., Wright, H.H. *et al.* (2009) 'Examination of tetrahydrobiopterin pathway genes in autism.' *Genes, Brain and Behavior, 8*(8): 753–757.

Schreck, K.A. (1997/1998) 'Preliminary analysis of sleep disorders in children with developmental disorders.' Doctoral dissertation, Ohio State University, 1997. *Dissertation Abstracts International, 58*, 3934.

Schreck, K.A. (2001) 'Behavioral treatments for sleep problems in autism: Empirically supported or just universally accepted?' *Behavioral Assessments, 16*(4): 265–278.

Schreck, K.A., Mulick, J.A. and Rojahn, J.A. (2003) 'Development of the Behavioral Evaluation of Disorders of Sleep Scale.' *Journal of Child and Family Studies, 12*(3): 349–360.

Schreck, K.A., Mulick, J.A. and Smith, A.F. (2004) 'Sleep problems as possible predictors of intensified symptoms of autism.' *Research in Developmental Disabilities, 25*: 57–66.

Schultz, S.T., Klonoff-Cohen, H.S., Wingard, D.L., Akshoomoff, N.A. *et al.* (2006) 'Breastfeeding, infant formula supplementation, and autistic disorder: The results of a parent survey.' *International Breastfeeding Journal, 1*: 16. doi:10.1186/1746-4358-1-16.

Schwartz, J.R.L. (2008) 'Modafinil in the treatment of excessive sleepiness.' *Drug Design, Development and Therapy, 2*: 71–85.

Seicean, A., Redline, S., Seicean, S., Kirchner, H.L. *et al.* (2007) 'Association between short sleeping hours and overweight in adolescents: Results from a US suburban high school survey.' *Sleep and Breathing, 11*: 285–293.

Senju, A., Maeda, M., Kikuchi, Y., Hasegawa, T. *et al.* (2007) 'Absence of contagious yawning in children with autism spectrum disorder.' *Biology Letters, 3*: 706–708.

Silber, M.H., Ehrenberg, B.L., Allen, R.P., Buchfuhrer, R.A. *et al.* (2004) 'An algorithm for the management of restless legs syndrome.' *Mayo Clinic Proceedings, 79*: 916–922.

Silvia, M. and Raffaele, F. (2010) 'Epidemiology and management of insomnia in children with autistic spectrum disorders.' *Pediatric Drugs, 12*(2): 75–84.

Simakajornboon, N., Gozal, D., Vlasic, V., Mack, C. *et al.* (2003) 'Periodic limb movements in sleep and iron status in children.' *Sleep, 26*: 735–738.

Simakajornboon, N., Kheirandish-Gozal, L., Gozal, D., Sharon, D. *et al.* (2006) 'A long term follow-up study of periodic limb movement disorders in children after iron therapy.' *Sleep, 29*(Suppl): A76.

Simard, V., Nielsen, T.A., Tremblay, R.E., Boivin, M. and Montplaisir, J.Y. (2008) 'Longitudinal study of bad dreams in preschool-aged children: Prevalence, demographic correlates, risk and protective factors.' *Sleep, 31*(1): 62–70.

Simonoff, E.A. and Stores, G. (1987) 'Controlled trial of trimeprazine tartrate for night waking.' *Archives of Disease in Childhood, 62*: 253–257.

Slifer, K.J., Avis, K.T. and Frutchey, R.A. (2008) ' Behavioral intervention to increase compliance with electroencephalographic procedures in children with developmental disabilities.' *Epilepsy and Behavior, 13*(1): 189–195.

Smith, G.C.S. and Pell, J.P. (2003) 'Parachute use to prevent death and major trauma related to gravitational challenge: Systematic review of randomised controlled trials.' *British Medical Journal, 327*: 1459–1461.

Smith, R., Ronald, J., Delaive, K., Walld, R. *et al.* (2002) 'What are obstructive sleep apnea patients being treated for prior to this diagnosis?' *Chest, 121*: 164–172.

Souders, M.C., Mason, T.B.A., Valladares, O., Bucan, M. *et al.* (2009) 'Sleep behaviors and sleep quality in children with autism spectrum disorders.' *Sleep, 32*(12): 1566–1578.

Spock, B. (1946) *The Commonsense Book of Baby and Child Care.* New York, NY: Duell, Sloane & Pearce.

Spock, B. revised and updated by Needleman, R. (2004) *The Commonsense Book of Baby and Child Care* (8th edn). New York, NY: Pocket Books.

Spoormaker, V.I. and Montgomery, P. (2008) 'Disturbed sleep in post-traumatic stress disorder: Secondary symptom or core feature?' *Sleep Medicine Reviews, 12*: 169–184.

Stepanova, I., Nevsimalova, S. and Hanusova, J. (2005) 'Rhythmic movement disorder in sleep persisting into childhood and adulthood.' *Sleep, 28*: 851–857.

Stickgold, R.J., Malia, A., Maguire, D., Roddenberry, D. and O'Connor, M. (2000) 'Replaying the game: Hypnagogic images in normals and amnesics.' *Science, 290*: 350–353.

Stores, G. (2001) 'Dramatic parasomnias.' *Journal of the Royal Society of Medicine, 94*(4): 173–176.

Strausz, T., Ahlberg, J., Lobbezoo, F., Restrepo, C.C. *et al.* (2010) 'Awareness of tooth grinding and clenching from adolescence to young adulthood: A nine-year follow-up.' *Journal of Oral Rehabilitation, 37*(7): 497–500.

Strean, W.B. (2009) 'Laughter prescription.' *Canadian Family Physician, 55*: 965–967.

Striegel-Moore, R.H., Dohm, F.A., Hook, J.M., Schreiber, G.B. *et al.* (2005) 'Night eating syndrome in young adult women: Prevalence and correlates.' *International Journal of Eating Disorders, 37*: 200–206.

Stroe, A.F., Roth, T., Jefferson, C., Hudgel, D.W. *et al.* (2010) 'Comparative levels of excessive daytime sleepiness in common medical disorders.' *Sleep Medicine, 11*(9): 890–896.

Stolz, S. and Aldrich, M. (1991) 'REM sleep behavior disorder associated with caffeine abuse.' *Sleep Research, 20*: 341.

Stunkard, A.J., Allison, K.C., Lundgren, J.D., Martino, N.S. *et al.* (2006) 'A paradigm for facilitating pharmacotherapy at a distance: Sertraline treatment of the night eating syndrome.' *Journal of Clinical Psychiatry, 67*(10): 1568–1572.

Su, C., Miao, J., Liu, Y., Liu, R. *et al.* (2009) 'Multiple forms of rhythmic movements in an adolescent boy with rhythmic movement disorder.' *Clinical Neurology and Neurosurgery, 111*: 896–899.

Szelenberger, W., Niemcewicz, S. and Dabrowska, A.J. (2005) 'Sleepwalking and night terrors: Psychopathological and psychophysiological correlates.' *International Review of Psychiatry, 17*: 263–270.

Tabandeh, H., Lockley, S.W., Buttery, R., Skene, D.J. *et al.* (1998) 'Disturbance of sleep in blindness.' *American Journal of Ophthalmology, 126*: 707–712.

Tachibana, N., Shinde, A., Ikeda, A., Akiguchi, I., Kimura, J. and Shibasaki, H. (1996) 'Supplementary motor area seizure resembling sleep disorder.' *Sleep, 19*: 811–816.

Tafti, M., Maret, S. and Dauvilliers, Y. (2005) 'Genes for normal sleep and sleep disorders.' *Annals of Medicine, 37*(8): 580–589.

Tager-Flusberg H. (1999) 'A psychological approach to understanding the social and language impairments in autism.' *International Review of Psychiatry, 11*(4): 325–334.

Tahmaz, L., Kibar, Y., Yildirim, I., Ceylan, S. and Dayanc, M. (2000) 'Combination therapy of imipramine with oxybutynin in children with enuresis nocturna.' *Urologia Internationalis, 65*(3): 135–139.

Tani, P., Lindberg, N., Joukamaa, M., Nieminen-von Wendt, T. *et al.* (2004) 'Sleep in young adults with Asperger syndrome.' *Neuropsychobiology, 50*: 147–152.

Tani, P., Lindberg, N., Nieminen-von Wendt, T., von Wendt, L. *et al.* (2003) 'Insomnia is a frequent finding in adults with Asperger syndrome.' *BMC Psychiatry, 3*. Available from www.biomedcentral.com/1471-244X/3/12, accessed 13 November 2013.

Taubes, G. (2007) *The Diet Delusion.* New York, NY: Alfred A. Knopf, Random House.

Taveras, E.M., Rifas-Shiman, S.L., Oken, E. Gunderson, E.P. and Gillman, M.W. (2008) 'Short sleep duration in infancy and risk of childhood overweight.' *Archives of Pediatric and Adolescent Medicine, 162*(4): 305–311.

Taylor, D.J., Mallory, L.J., Lichstein, K.L., Durrence, H.H. *et al.* (2007) 'Comorbidity of chronic insomnia with medical problems.' *Sleep, 30*: 213–218.

Taylor, J.H. (ed.) (1932) *Selected Writings of John Hughlings Jackson.* London: Hodder and Stoughton.

Thannickal, T.C., Nienhuis, R. and Siegel, J.M. (2009) 'Localized loss of hypocretin (orexin) cells in narcolepsy without cataplexy.' *Sleep, 32*(8): 993–998.

Thirumalai, S., Shubin, R. and Robinson, R. (2002) 'Rapid eye movement sleep behavior disorder in children with autism.' *Journal of Child Neurology, 17*(3): 173–178.

Thompson, M.D., Comings, D.E., Abu-Ghazalah, R., Jereseh, Y. *et al.* (2004) 'Variants of the orexin2/hcrt2 receptor gene identified in patients with excessive daytime sleepiness and patients with Tourette's syndrome comorbidity.' *American Journal of Medical Genetics B: Neuropsychiatric Genetics, 129B*(1): 69–75.

Thompson, S.B.N. (2010) 'The dawn of the yawn: Is yawning a warning? Linking neurological disorders.' *Medical Hypotheses, 75*: 630–633.

Thorburn, P.T. and Riha, R.L. (2010) 'Skin disorders and sleep in adults: Where is the evidence?' *Sleep Medicine Reviews, 14*: 351–358.

Tinuper, P., Provini, F., Bisulli, F., Vignatelli, L. *et al.* (2007) 'Movement disorders in sleep: Guidelines for differentiating epileptic from non-epileptic motor phenomena arising from sleep.' *Sleep Medicine Reviews, 11*: 255–267.

Toro, R., Konyukh, M., Delorme, R., Leblond, C. *et al.* (2010) 'Key role for gene dosage and synaptic homeostasis in autism spectrum disorders.' *Trends in Genetics, 20*: 1–10. doi:10.1016/j.tig.2010.05.007.

Tractenberg, R.E. and Singer, C.M. (2007) 'Sleep and sleep disturbance: From genes to dreams.' *Cellular and Molecular Life Sciences, 64*: 1171–1173.

Trachtman, J.N. (2010) 'Vision and the hypothalamus.' Optometry, 81: 100–115.

Trenell, M.I., Marshall, N.S. and Rogers N.L. (2007) 'Sleep and metabolic control: Waking to a problem?' *Clinical and Experimental Pharmacology and Physiology, 34*(1): 1–9.

Trenkwalder, C., Hening, W.A., Montagna, P. *et al.* (2008) 'Treatment of restless legs syndrome: An evidence-based review and implications for clinical practice.' *Movement Disorders, 23*: 2267–2302.

Tudor, M.E., Hoffman, C.D. and Sweeney, D.P. (2012) 'Children with autism sleep problems and symptom severity.' *Focus on Autism and Other Developmental Disabilities, 27*(4): 254–262.

Valenti, G., Laera, A., Gouraud, S., Pace, G. *et al.* (2002) 'Low-calcium diet in hypercalciuric enuretic children restores AQP2 excretion and improves clinical symptoms.' *American Journal of Physiology – Renal Fluid & Electrolyte Physiology, 283*(5): F895–F903.

Vallieres, A., Morin, C.M. and Guay, B. (2005) 'Sequential combinations of drug and cognitive behavioural therapy for chronic insomnia: An exploratory study.' *Behaviour Research and Therapy, 43*: 1611–1630.

Van Cauter, E. and Knutson, K.L. (2008) 'Sleep and the epidemic of obesity in children and adults.' *European Journal of Endocrinology, 159*: S59–S66.

Van de Walle, J., Stockner, M., Raes, A. and Nørgaard, J.P. (2007) 'Desmopressin 30 years in clinical use: A safety review.' *Current Drug Safety, 2*(3): 232–238.

Van de Walle, J., Van Herzeele, C. and Raes, A. (2010) 'Is there still a role for desmopressin in children with primary monosymptomatic nocturnal enuresis?: A focus on safety issues.' *Drug Safety, 33*(4): 261–271.

Varan, B., Saatci, U., Ozen, S., Bakkaloglu, A. and Besbas, N. (1996) 'Efficacy of oxybutynin, pseudoephedrine and indomethacin in the treatment of primary nocturnal enuresis.' *Turkish Journal of Pediatrics, 38*(2): 155–159.

Varni, J.W. (1992) *Clinical Behavioral Pediatrics: An Interdisciplinary Biobehavioral Approach.* Princeton, NJ: Prentice-Hall.

Vernet, C. and Arnulf, I. (2009) 'Idiopathic hypersomnia with and without long sleep time: A controlled series of 75 patients.' *Sleep, 32*(6): 753–759.

Vessey, J.A., Carlson, K.L. and McGill, J. (1994) 'Use of distraction with children during an acute pain experience.' *Nursing Research, 43*(6): 369–372.

Vetrugno, R., Manconi, M., Ferini-Strambi, L., Provini, F. *et al.* (2006) 'Nocturnal eating: Sleep-related eating disorder or night eating syndrome? A videopolysomnographic study.' *Sleep, 29*: 949–954.

Vorona, R.D. and Ware, J.C. (2002) 'Exacerbation of REM sleep behavior disorder by chocolate ingestion: A case report.' *Sleep Medicine, 3*: 365–367.

Wagner, M.H. and Berry, R.B. (2007) 'An obese female with Prader-Willi syndrome and daytime sleepiness.' *Journal of Clinical Sleep Medicine, 3*(6): 645–647.

Walters, A.S., Mandelbaum, D.E., Lewin, D.S., Kugler, S. *et al.* (2000) 'Dopaminergic therapy in children with restless legs/periodic limb movements in sleep and ADHD, Dopaminergic Therapy Study Group.' *Pediatric Neurology, 22*: 182–186.

Walters, A.S., Silvestri, R., Zucconi, M., Chandrashekariah, R. and Konofal, E. (2008) 'Review of the possible relationship and hypothetical links between attention deficit hyperactivity disorder (ADHD) and the simple sleep related movement disorders, parasomnias, hypersomnias, and circadian rhythm disorders.' *Journal of Clinical Sleep Medicine, 4*(6): 591–600.

Wassink, T.H., Piven, J., Vieland, V.J., Jenkins, L. *et al.* (2005) 'Evaluation of the chromosome 2q37.3 gene CENTG2 as an autism susceptibility gene.' *American Journal of Medical Genetics Part B Neuropsychiatric Genetics, 136*: 36–44.

Watts, D.J. (2011) *Everything Is Obvious*– How Common Sense Fails (*once you know the answer).* New York, NY: Random House.

Weaver, T.E. (2001) 'Outcome measurement in sleep medicine practice and research. Part 1: Assessment of symptoms, subjective and objective daytime sleepiness, health-related quality of life and functional status.' *Sleep Medicine Reviews, 5*(2): 103–128.

Weidong, W., Fang, W., Yang, Z., Menghan, L. and Xueyu, L. (2009) 'Two patients with narcolepsy treated by hypnotic psychotherapy.' *Sleep Medicine, 10*: 1167–1169.

Weiss, L.A., Kosova, G., Delahanty, R.J., Jiang, L. *et al.* (2006) 'Variation in ITGB3 is associated with whole-blood serotonin level and autism susceptibility.' *European Journal of Human Genetics, 76*: 1050–1056.

Werner, H., LeBourgeois, M.K., Geiger, A. and Jenni, O.G. (2009) 'Assessment of chronotype in four- to eleven-year-old children: Reliability and validity of the Children's Chronotype Questionnaire (CCTQ).' *Chronobiology International, 26*(5): 992–1014.

Whelan-Goodinson, R., Ponsford, J., Johnston, L. and Grant, F. (2009) 'Psychiatric disorders following traumatic brain injury: their nature and frequency.' *Journal of Head Trauma Rehabilitation, 24*(5): 324–332.

Widmalm, S.E., Christiansen, R.L. and Gunn, S.M. (1995) 'Oral parafunctions as temporomandibular disorder risk factors in children.' *Cranio: The Journal of Craniomandibular Practice, 13*(4): 242–246.

Wietske, R., Kox, D., den Herder, C., van Tintern, H. and de Vries, N. (2007) 'One stage multilevel surgery (uvulopalatopharyngoplasty, hyoid suspension, radiofrequent ablation of the tongue base with/without genioglossus advancement), in obstructive sleep apnea syndrome.' *European Archives of Oto-Rhino-Laryngology, 264*(4): 439–444.

Wimpory, D., Nicholas, B. and Nash S. (2002) 'Social timing, clock genes and autism: A new hypothesis.' *Journal of Intellectual Disability Research, 46*(4): 352–358.

Wood, J.J., Piacentini, J.C., Southam-Gerow, M. and Sigman, M. (2006) 'Family cognitive behavioral therapy for child anxiety disorders.' *Journal of the American Academy of Child and Adolescent Psychiatry, 45*(3): 314–321.

Wright, A. (2008) 'Evidence-based assessment and management of childhood enuresis.' *Paediatrics and Child Health, 18*(12): 561–567.

Wright, B., Sims, D., Smart, S., Alwazeer, A. *et al.* (2011) 'Melatonin versus placebo in children with autism spectrum conditions and severe sleep problems not amenable to behaviour management strategies: A randomized controlled crossover trial.' *Journal of Autism and Developmental Disorders, 41*(2): 175–184.

Wulff, K., Porcheret, K., Cussans, E. and Foster, R.G. (2009) 'Sleep and circadian rhythm disturbances: Multiple genes and multiple phenotypes.' *Current Opinion in Genetics and Development, 19*: 237–246.

Yang, S., Liu, A., Weidenhammer, A., Cooksey, R.C. *et al.* (2009) 'The role of mPer2 clock gene in glucocorticoid and feeding rhythms.' *Endocrinology, 150:* 2153–2160.

Yeung, C.K., Sreedhar, B., Sihoe, J.D., Sit, F.K. and Lau, J. (2006) 'Differences in characteristics of nocturnal enuresis between children and adolescents: A critical appraisal from a large epidemiological study.' *British Journal of Urology International, 97:* 1069–1073.

Yoo, S-S., Gujar, N., Hu, P., Jolesz, F.A. and Walker, M.P. (2007) 'The human emotional brain without sleep – a prefrontal amygdala disconnect.' *Current Biology, 17*(20): R877–R878.

Yu-lian, X., Xiao-yun, L. and Chun-hua, D. (2002) 'Treatment observations and results of 50 cases of pediatric enuresis with Yi Niao Ling Fang [in Chinese].' *Xin Zhong Yi (New Chinese Medicine), 12:* 27–28. (Translation by R. Helmer available from: www.goldenneedleonline.com/blog/2009/08/09/treatment-observations-results-of-50-cases-of-pediatric-enuresis-with-yi-niao-ling-fang-effective, accessed 13 November 2013.)

Zee, P.C. and Manthena, P. (2007) 'The brain's master circadian clock: Implications and opportunities for therapy of sleep disorders.' *Sleep Medicine Reviews, 11:* 59–70.

Zeitzer, J.M., Dijk, D.J., Kronauer, R.E., Brown, E.N. and Czeisler, C.A. (2000) 'Sensitivity of the human circadian pacemaker to nocturnal light: Melatonin phase resetting and suppression.' *Journal of Physiology, 526*(3): 695–702.

Zeitzer, J.M., Nishino, S. and Mignot, E. (2006) 'The neurobiology of hypocretins (orexins), narcolepsy and related therapeutic interventions.' *Trends in Pharmacological Sciences, 27*(7): 368–374.

Zelikovsky, N., Rodrigue, J.R., Gidycz, C.A. and Davis, M.A. (2000) 'Cognitive behavioral and behavioral interventions help young children cope during a voiding cystourethrogram.' *Journal of Pediatric Psychology, 25*(8): 535–543.

Zhao, Q., Sherrill, D.L., Goodwin, J.L. and Quan, S.F. (2008) 'Association between sleep disordered breathing and behavior in school-aged children: The Tucson Children's Assessment of Sleep Apnea Study.' *Open Epidemiology Journal, 1:* 1–9.

Zhdanova, I.V., Wurtman, R.J. and Wagstaff, J. (1999) 'Effects of a low dose of melatonin on sleep in children with Angelman syndrome.' *Journal of Pediatric Endocrinology and Metabolism, 12*(1): 57–67.

FURTHER READING

After getting this far, some people may wish to read further on ASD, on sleep and on issues around sleep difficulties. For those of you who do, here are some suggestions for further exploration. I do not endorse all of the views that can be found in every one of the following books, but have provided various suggestions of books to help people who want to read and learn more on these issues, but might not be able to access some of the source journal articles I have drawn on.

Accessible general books on autistic spectrum disorders

Attwood, T. and Isaacs, P. (2013) *A Pocket Size Practical Guide for Parents, Professionals and People on The Autistic Spectrum.* Truro: Chipmunkapublishing.

Baron-Cohen, S. (2009) *Autism: The Facts.* Oxford: Oxford University Press.

Boucher, J. (2008) *The Autistic Spectrum: Characteristics, Causes and Practical Issues.* London: SAGE Publications.

Coplan, J. (2009) *Making Sense of Autistic Spectrum Disorders: Create the Brightest Future for Your Child with the Best Treatment Options.* New York: Bantam Books.

Frith, U. (2008) *Autism: A Very Short Introduction.* Oxford: Oxford University Press.

Sicile-Kira, C. (2003) *Autism Spectrum Disorders: The Complete Guide.* London: Vermillion.

Wing, L. (2003) *The Autistic Spectrum* (new updated edition). London: Constable & Robinson.

Accessible general books on sleep

Hobson, J.A. (1988) *The Dreaming Brain.* New York: Basic Books.

Horne, J. (2006) *Sleepfaring: A Journey through the Science of Sleep.* Oxford: Oxford University Press.

Jouvet, M. (2008) *The Paradox of Sleep: The Castle of Dreams.* Cambridge, MA: MIT Press.

Martin, P. (2002) *Counting Sheep: The Science and Pleasures of Sleep and Dreams.* London: HarperCollins.

Oswald, I. (1966) *Sleep.* Harmondsworth: Penguin.

Randall, D.K. (2012) *Dreamland: Adventures in the Strange Science of Sleep.* New York: W.W. Norton.

Roenneberg, T. (2012) *Internal Time: Chronotypes, Social Jet Lag, and Why You're So Tired.* Boston, MA: Harvard University Press.

Accessible general books on sleep problems and sleep disorders

Carranza, C. (2004) *Banishing Night Terrors and Nightmares.* London: Kensington Books.

Daymond, K. (2001) *The 'Parentalk' Guide to Sleep.* London: Hodder & Stoughton.

Douglas, J. and Richman, N. (1988) *My Child Won't Sleep.* Harmondsworth: Penguin.

Durand, M.V. (1997) *Sleep Better! Guide to Improving Sleep for Children with Special Needs.* Baltimore, MD: Paul H. Brookes.

Durand, M.V. (2008a) *When Children Don't Sleep Well: Interventions for Pediatric Sleep Disorders Therapist Guide (Treatments that Work).* Oxford: Oxford University Press.

Durand, M.V. (2008b) *When Children Don't Sleep Well: Interventions for Pediatric Sleep Disorders Parent Workbook (Treatments that Work).* Oxford: Oxford University Press.

Epstein, L. and Mardon, S. (2006) *The Harvard Medical School Guide to a Good Night's Sleep.* New York: McGraw-Hill.

Espie, C.A. (2006) *Overcoming Insomnia and Sleep Problems: A Self-Help Guide Using Cognitive Behavioral Techniques.* London: Constable and Robinson.

Ferber, R. (1985) *Solve Your Child's Sleep Problems.* New York: Simon and Schuster.

Flanagan, O.J. (2001) *Dreaming Souls: Sleep, Dreams and the Evolution of the Conscious Mind.* New York: Oxford University Press.

Haslam, D. (1992) *Sleepless Children: A Handbook for Parents.* London: Piatkus.

Hirshkowitz, M. and Smith, P.B. (2004) *Sleep Disorders for Dummies.* Hoboken, NJ: Wiley.

Hollyer, B. (2002) *Sleep: The Easy Way to Peaceful Nights.* London: Cassell.

Karp, H. (2012) *The Happiest Baby Guide to Great Sleep: Simple Solutions for Kids from Birth to 5 Years.* New York: William Morrow (HarperCollins).

Mansbach, A. (2011) *Go the Fuck to Sleep.* New York: Akashik Books.

Margo, S. (2008) *The Good Sleep Guide.* London: Vermillion.

Morrisroe, P. (2010) *Wide Awake.* New York: Spiegel & Grau.

Pantley, E. (2002) *The No-Cry Sleep Solution: Gentle Ways to Help Your Baby Sleep Through the Night.* Chicago, IL: McGraw-Hill.

Stores, G. (2009a) *The Facts: Sleep Problems in Children and Adolescents.* Oxford: Oxford University Press.

Stores, G. (2009b) *Insomnia and Other Adult Sleep Problems: The Facts.* Oxford: Oxford University Press.

Wiedman, J. (1998) *Desperately Seeking Snoozing: The Insomnia Cure from Awake to Zzzz.* Madison, WI: University of Wisconsin Press.

Wiley, T.S. and Formby, B. (2000) *Lights Out: Sleep Sugar and Survival.* New York: Simon & Schuster.

Wilson, S. and Nutt D. (2008) *Sleep Disorders* (Oxford Psychiatry Library). Oxford: Oxford University Press.

RESOURCES

Sleep associations and web resources

There are a large number of National and International Sleep Associations. Many of these can put you in touch with support groups and provide information on local therapists, clinics and other resources. Contact details for some of the main ones are provided below.

American Academy of Sleep Medicine
2510 North Frontage Road
Darien, IL 60561
USA
Tel: (630) 737-9700
Fax: (630) 737-9790
Email: inquiries@aasmnet.org
Website: www.aasmnet.org

American Sleep Apnea Association
6856 Eastern Avenue, NW, Suite 203
Washington, DC 20012
USA
Tel: (202) 293-3650
Fax: (202) 293-3656
Website: www.sleepapnea.org

American Sleep Association
Website: www.sleepassociation.org

Associated Professional Sleep Societies, LLC
2510 North Frontage Road
Darien, IL 60561
USA
Tel: (630) 737-9700
Fax: (630) 737-9789
Website: www.sleepmeeting.org

British Sleep Society
PO Box 247
Colne
Huntingdon PE28 3UZ
England
Email: enquiries@sleeping.org.uk
Website: www.neuronic.com/british.htm

British Snoring & Sleep Apnoea Association
Castle Court, 41 London Road
Reigate
Surrey RH2 9RJ
England
Tel: 01737 245638
Email: info@britishsnoring.co.uk
Website: www.britishsnoring.co.uk

Edinburgh Sleep Centre
13 Heriot Row
Edinburgh EH3 6HP
Scotland
Fax: 0131 524 9730
Website: www.edinburghsleepcentre.com

Enuresis Resource and Information Centre (ERIC)
34 Old School House, Britannia Road
Kingswood
Bristol BS15 8DB
England
Helpline: 0845 370 8008 (10am–4pm weekdays)
Tel: 0845 370 8008
Email: info@eric.org.uk
Website: www.eric.org.uk

London Sleep Centre
137 Harley Street
London W1G 6BF
England
Tel: 020 7725 0523
Email: info@londonsleepcentre.com
Website: www.londonsleepcentre.com

Narcolepsy Association UK (UKAN)
PO Box 13842
Penicuik EH26 8WX
Scotland
Tel: 0845 4500 394
Email: info@narcolepsy.org.uk
Website: www.narcolepsy.org.uk

Narcolepsy Network
110 Ripple Lane
North Kingstown, RI 02852
USA
Toll-free: (888) 292-6522
Tel: (401) 667-2523
Fax: (401) 633-6567
Website: www.narcolepsynetwork.org

National Center on Sleep Disorders Research
National Heart, Lung, and Blood Institute, NIH
6701 Rockledge Drive
Bethesda, MD 20892
USA
Tel: 301-435-0199
Fax: 301-480-3451
Website: http://rover.nhlbi.nih.gov/about/ncsdr

National Foundation for Sleep and Related Disorders in Children (NFSRDC)
4200 W. Peterson, Suite 109
Chicago, IL 60646
USA
Tel: (708) 971-1086
Fax: (312) 434-5311

National Sleep Foundation
1522 K Street, NW, Suite 500
Washington, DC 20005
USA
Tel: (202) 347-3471
Fax: (202) 347-3472
Email: nsf@sleepfoundation.org
Website: www.sleepfoundation.org

Restless Legs Syndrome Foundation (now Willis-Ekbom Disease Foundation)
1610 14th St NW Rochester, Suite 300
Rochester, MN   55902-2985
USA
Tel: 507-287-6465
Email: rlsfoundation@rls.org
Website: www.rls.org

Sleep Apnoea Trust Association (SATA)
12A Bakers Place
Kingston
Oxfordshire OX39 4SW
England
Tel: 0845 60 60 685
Website: www.sleep-apnoea-trust.org

Sleep Matters Helpline
PO Box 3087
London W4 4ZP
England
Tel: 020 8994 9874 (6pm–8pm daily)
Email: info@medicaladvisoryservice.org.uk
Website: www.medicaladvisoryservice.org.uk

Sleep Research Society
2510 North Frontage Road
Darien, IL 60561
USA
Tel: (630) 737-9702
Website: www.sleepresearchsociety.org

Sleep Scotland
8 Hope Park Square
Edinburgh EH8 9NW
Scotland
Tel: 0131 651 1392
Fax: 0131 651 1391
Website: www.sleepscotland.org

Stanford Sleep and Dreams
Website: www.end-your-sleep-deprivation.com/sleep-and-dreams.html

World Sleep Federation: World Federation of Sleep Research and Sleep Medicine Societies
Website: www.wfsrsms.org

Melatonin testing

Testing for circadian differences in melatonin levels is not a routine party of clinical investigation in the UK or in many US clinics. Salivary testing is the easiest and least invasive method of assessment and can be obtained from Genova Diagnostics in Europe and North America (comprehensive melatonin profile, saliva).

Genova Diagnostics
63 Zillicoa Street
Asheville, NC 28801
USA
Tel: 800-522-4762

Genova Diagnostics Europe Headquarters
Parkgate House, 356 West Barnes Lane
New Malden
Surrey KT3 6NB
England
Tel: 020 8336 7750

General products to aid sleep

Light Therapy Products
5865 Neal Avenue North, Suite 153
Stillwater MN, Maryland 55082
USA
Website: www.lighttherapyproducts.com
This company markets a range of lighting products, and in addition a variety of other products including sleep CDs, hypoallergenic bedding and blackout kits.

Devices to treat obstructive sleep apnoea

Various devices are available that are aimed at keeping the airway open during sleep and reduce/eliminate snoring. A representative range of companies offering such devices follows. No specific endorsement is made of any of these products and those interested are encouraged to seek information on any device and its effectiveness from the manufacturer/distributor before considering its use.

Ripsnore
PO Box 16283
City East, Brisbane Q 4002
Australia
Tel: 0410-843-498

PO Box 225065
San Francisco, CA 94122-5065
USA
Tel: (+1) 415-699-0264

PO Box 40025
Ottawa, ON K1V 0W8
Canada
Tel: (+1) 613-355-6496

PO Box 64965
London SW19 9BL
England
Tel: 07794 489044
Website: www.ripsnore.com

SleepPro
MEDiTAS Ltd
PO Box 567
Winchester
Hampshire SO23 2HJ
England
Tel: 01962 761 831
Website: www.sleeppro.com

Snorban
Snoring Relief Labs, Inc.
4007 Pretense Ct
Fair Oaks, CA 95628
USA
Tel: (916) 966-5026
Website: www.snorban.com

Snoremender
Sleep Well Enjoy Life Ltd
12 Station Road
Eckington
Sheffield S21 4FX
England

TheraSnore
Distar UK Ltd
Manor Farm House, Main Street
Gamston
Nottingham NG2 6NN
England
Tel: 0115 969 64 29
Website: www.therasnore.co.uk

Enuresis (bedwetting) alarms

Enuresis alarms are readily available and can be purchased for home use. A wide range of such alarms is now available. I make no specific endorsement, either for the efficacy or safety of any of these products. Those interested are encouraged to seek information on devices and their effectiveness from the manufacturer/distributor before considering their use.

Europe

Astric
Astric Medical
148 Lewes Road
Brighton
Sussex BN2 3LG
England
Tel: 01273 608 319
Email: astricmed@aol.com

Drinite
Drinite Vibrawake
Rodger Wireless Bedwetting Alarm System
Dri-Nites
199 Aston Clinton Road
Aylesbury
Bucks HP22 5AD
England
Tel: 01296 631118
Website: www.dri-nites.co.uk

Enurad
ENURAD® AB
Östra Trädal 310
S-442 94 Ytterby
Sweden
Tel: +46 (0)303 58400
Email: info@enurad.com
Website: http://enurad.com

Malem
Malem Medical
10 Willow Holt
Lowdham
Nottingham NG14 7EJ
England
Tel: 0115 966 4440
Website: www.malemmedical.com

Noppy Bed-Wetting Eneuresis Alarm
Rehan Electronics Ltd
Brunswick Row
Aughrim Road
Carnew
County Wicklow
Republic of Ireland
Tel: 00353 53 9426742
Website: www.rehanelectronics.com

Petit Enuresis Alarm
Nottingham Rehab Supplies (NRS)
Clinitron House, Excelsior Road
Ashby de la Zouch
Leicestershire LE65 1JG
England
Tel: 0845 121 8111
Website: www.nrs-uk.co.uk

Various models are available from:

Living Made Easy
Disabled Living Foundation
380–384 Harrow Road
London W9 2HU
England
Helpline: 0845 130 9177

North America

Website with many links: www.xmarks.com/site/www.kidshealth.org/
parent/general/sleep/enuresis.html

DRI Sleeper
AMG Medical
8505 Dalton
Montreal
Quebec H4T 1V5
Canada
Tel: 514-737-5251
Website: www.amgmedical.com

NiteTrain-r
Koregon Enterprises Inc.
9735 SW Sunshine Court, Suite 100
Beaverton, OR 97005
USA
Tel: (800) 544-4240
Website: www.nitetrain-r.com

Nytone
Nytone Inc.
2424 S. 900 W.
Salt Lake City, UT 84119
USA
Tel: (801) 973 4090
Website: www.nytone.com

Potty Pager
Ideas for Living Inc.
1285 N. Cedarbrook Road
Boulder, CO 80394
USA
Tel: (800) 497-6573

Sleep Dry Alarm
Starchild Labs
PO Box 3497
57 Tierra Cielo Lane
Santa Barbara, CA 93105
USA
Tel: (805) 564-7194
Website: www.sleepdry.com/index.html

Wet-Stop 3 Alarm
PottyMD
6800 Baum Dr. Bldg. A
Knoxville
TN 37919
USA
Tel: 1-877-768-8963
Website: www.pottymd.com/?osCsid=c0ec066fe086b36c9f89e299b5c64
292

Rest of world

DRI Sleeper
Anzacare Ltd
120 Princess Drive
Nelson
New Zealand
Tel (US): (877) 331 2768
Tel (NZ): 4-3-5489655
Website: www.dri-sleeper.com

F-Star Infant Bed-wetting Alarm
PandaWill
Room 405, Eastwing, Huamei Building
ZhenXing Road
518000 Shenzhen
Guandong
China
Tel: 0086 755 83650148
Website: www.pandawill.com/baby-urine-bed-wetting-enuresis-alarm-p56
145.html

Epilepsy sensors

Night-time seizures are not uncommon and a number of commercial systems are now available to monitor nocturnal seizure activity. These are typically triggered by changes in movement or breathing. In many areas such devices may be available through local health services or epilepsy charities, which should be explored before any consideration is given to purchasing such equipment, which is likely to be expensive and complex to set up.

Bedside Monitor (P154); Advanced Bedside Monitor (P139)
Alert It
iTs Designs (Alert-it Alarms)
Atherstone House, Merry Lees Industrial Estate
Desford LE9 9FE
England
Tel: 0845 217 9951
Website: www.alert-it.co.uk

Emfit Nocturnal Tonic-Clonic Seizure Monitor
Emfit Ltd
Konttisentie 8 B
Vaajakoski FI-40800
Finland
Tel: 358 14 332 9000
Website: www.emfit.com

Emfit, Corp.
P.O. Box 342394
Austin, TX 78734
USA
Tel: (512) 266-6950
Website: www.emfit.com

MedPage (various models)
Easylink UK
3 Melbourne House, Corby Gate Business Park
Priors Haw Road
Corby
Northants NN17 5JG
England
Tel: 01536 264 869
Website: www.easylinkuk.co.uk

Sensalert EP200 Epilepsy Monitor
Sensorium Ltd
9 Netherton Broad Street
Dunfermline
Fife KY12 7DS
Scotland
Tel: 01383 720 600
Website: www.sensorium.co.uk

If the alarm is for a child, under 18 years of age, with uncontrolled epilepsy, they may qualify for a free bed alarm, generously donated through the Muir Maxwell Trust. Your paediatric neurologist or paediatric epilepsy nurse will have details and is able to refer you; alternatively, contact the Trust enquiries line on their website (www.muirmaxwelltrust.com), or write to them for an application form.

The Muir Maxwell Trust
First Floor, Suite 12, Stuart House
Eskmills, Musselburgh
East Lothian EH21 7PB
Scotland

Additional web-based resources

William C. Dement (2008) 'TechTalk' lecture to Google: 'The Role of Sleep in Achieving Happiness at Google', September: www.sleepquest.com/sq_dement.shtml

The Mayo clinic has a good open access website that provides general information on a range of sleep disorders: www.mayoclinic.com/health/search/search

Research Autism, a UK Charity which focuses on ASD research, has a large amount of material accessible online about sleep in ASD and a range of possible treatments. They are supporting a sleep database for problems in ASD being developed by Keele University.

Adam House, 1 Fitzroy Square
London W1T 5HE
Tel. 020 3490 3091
Website: www.researchautism.net/pages/welcome/home.ikml

The Royal College of Psychiatry has a downloadable leaflet on childhood sleep problems: www.rcpsych.ac.uk/healthadvice/parentsandyouthinfo/parents carers/sleepproblems.aspx

Appendix 1
THE MAIN MEDICATIONS
USED IN SLEEP DISORDERS
THEIR PRIMARY USES AND POSSIBLE ISSUES

(For referencing, see: Aitken 2011.)

Medication	Primary use in sleep problems	Possible issues
Alimemazine tartrate aka Trimeprazine tartrate	Night-waking	Irregular heart rate; slowed breathing
Aripiprazole	To induce tiredness (Use for sleep problems is off-label and there are no published studies on its use)	Weight gain, extrapyramidal symptoms, restlessness, sedation, headache, nausea
Clonidine	To induce tiredness	Clonidine can cause raised and decreased blood pressure
Chloral hydrate	To induce tiredness	Stomach upset, irregular heart rate and skin problems. On stopping, physical withdrawal effects, hallucinations, delusions and visual disturbances
Desmopressin acetate	Bedwetting	Hyponatraemia
Diphenhydramine	To induce tiredness (use for sleep problems is off-label and there are no published studies on its use)	Can have paradoxical effects in infants from excitation to seizures and death
Fluoxetine	Has been used to treat isolated sleep paralysis. More commonly a cause of sleep problems	Stopping fluoxetine can cause RLS and PLMS

Medication	Primary use in sleep problems	Possible issues
Hydroxyzine	Insomnia (primarily used for control of anxiety and as an antihistamine. Use for sleep problems is off-label and there are no published studies on its use)	Daytime drowsiness; paradoxical hyperactivity; cardiac toxicity when used in excess
Melatonin	Improves getting to sleep	Generally well tolerated with few reported side-effects
Mianserin (replaced by mirtazapine)	Night-time enuresis	Less effective than alternatives like desmopressin
Modafinil	Narcolepsy, EDS and associated memory and attentional problems	Stevens-Johnson syndrome (US Food and Drug Administration or FDA)
Prazosin	Nightmares and other sleep effects of PTSD	Currently used only for hypertension in children as it lowers blood pressure
Risperidone	To induce tiredness (FDA approved for treatment of irritability in ASD. Use for sleep problems is off-label and there are no published studies on its use)	Tiredness and weight gain are the main reasons for discontinuing use
Ramelteon	As for melatonin	Occasionally this can cause the production of breast milk by both males and females
Sodium oxybate	Treatment of narcolepsy (FDA approved for the management of narcolepsy-cataplexy)	Physical dependence; can cause psychosis, seizures and suicidal thoughts on withdrawal

Appendix 2
SUMMARY TABLE ON NON-PHARMACOLOGICAL APPROACHES

Approach	Strength of evidence base	Used for	Availability	Contra-indications
Acupuncture	Weak	No specific studies on use for sleep. Some reported improvements in people treated for other issues. One child study on use in cerebral palsy	Variable	None reported
Aromatherapy	Weak	One good feasibility study on its use. Nothing on clinical benefit	Widely available	Pregnancy, hypertension, thrombosis
Behavioural approaches	Good	See information on specific sleep problems	Widely available	None reported
Biofeedback	Good for nocturnal enuresis; limited for other conditions	Nocturnal enuresis; nocturnal seizures; insomnia	Limited	None reported
Buchu (South African herbal)	Anecdotal	Nocturnal enuresis	Limited	Unclear

Approach	Strength of evidence base	Used for	Availability	Contra-indications
Chinese herbal	No RCT evidence	Insomnia, nocturnal enuresis, night terrors	Widely available	See information on specific herbs and sleep problems
Chiropractics	Limited	Single case studies on sleep problems. One clinical trial on nocturnal enuresis. One single case study in ASD	Widely available	None reported
Cognitive-behavioural approaches	Good	Insomnia	Widely available	None reported
Dietary interventions	Weak	Secondary evidence of beneficial effects in treatment for other reasons – ADHD, ASD	Widely available	See: Aitken (2008)
Exercise	Limited	Insomnia RCT (adult), snoring RCT (child)	Widely	None reported
Homeopathy	Limited – one RCT	Insomnia	Widely available	Pregnancy
Hypnosis	Fair but no RCT data	Insomnia and parasomnias	Variable	Psychosis, schizophrenia, epilepsy, depression
Japanese Kampo herbal medicine	Limited	Nocturnal enuresis, insomnia, night sweats	Limited outside Japan	See information on specific herbs and combinations
Light therapy	Good	Sleep phase syndromes	Variable	None reported
Massage	Fair	Settling to sleep	Widely available	None

Meditation	Limited	Difficulty with getting to sleep	Widely available	None reported
Traditional Mexican herbal treatments	Anecdotal	'Sleep problems'	Limited outside North America	Not known
Prescription medications	Good	See information above and sections on specific sleep problems	Widely available	Varies dependent on medication
Psychotherapy (analytic)	Limited	Unclear	Limited	Not used for this purpose
Relaxation	Fair	Insomnia and as part of a combined approach for most other sleep difficulties	Widely available	None reported
'Western' herbal treatments	Variable	Better evidence for stimulant herbs on tiredness than sedative herbs for insomnia but some support for both	Widely: largely unregulated	See information on specific herbs
Yoga	Limited	Improved sleep quality	Widely available	None

Appendix 3
WESTERN HERBS USED
IN SLEEP DISORDERS

(For referencing, see: Aitken 2011.)

Herb/extract	Primary use in sleep problems	Possible issues
Sedative		
Californian poppy	Used in combination with other herbs to reduce anxiety/agitation	Limited data
Chamomile	Insomnia	Idiosyncratic reactions (rare)
Ginseng	Reduce response to stress	Bizarre manic behaviour (rare)
Hops	Mildly sedative? Supporting evidence lacking	No evidence of physiological effect
Kava kava	Helps to produce a sense of calm and relaxation	Some concerns over liver toxicity (rare)
Lemon balm	Mildly calming and sedative	None of note
Immature oat seeds	Mildly sedative	No evidence of any significant positive or negative effects
Passionflower	Treatment of insomnia	Generally considered safe
Skullcap	Mildly sedative	Limited data
St John's Wort	General calming and antidepressant	Overall problem rate similar to placebo. Some cases reported of agitated psychotic behaviour (rare)
Valerian	General disturbance of sleep and insomnia	Safe but limited data on efficacy

Stimulant		
Caffeine	Improves vigilance and concentration	Psychotic and cardiovascular reactions and some fatalities at high doses
Ephedra	Stimulant	Seizures. Currently banned in the USA and now prescription only in the UK
Yohimbine	Increases attention and activity level	Nausea, vomiting, abdominal pain

Appendix 4
CHINESE HERBS USED IN SLEEP DISORDERS
PRIMARY USES AND POSSIBLE ISSUES

(For further information and referencing, see: Aitken 2012.)

Herb/ extract	Primary use in sleep problems	Possible issues
Baijianggen	Difficulty sleeping – insomnia (as for valerian)	See under Valerian in previous section
Baiziren	Insomnia, motor restlessness, night sweats	Variation in constituents of different types
Banxia	Insomnia	Contains ephedrine
Chaihu	Insomnia (usually in combination – see Da-Chai-Hu-Tang and Xiao-Chai-Hu-Tang below)	No safety information when used singly. Some concerns over liver toxicity from Da-Chai-Hu-Tang and Xiao-Chai-Hu-Tang which contain chaihu
Chuanxiong	Insomnia	None noted. Overdose can induce vomiting and dizziness
Danggui	Insomnia	Only evaluation in treatment of menopausal sleep problems
Danshen	Problems sleeping due to overarousal	Counteracts blood thinning medications like warfarin. Interferes with Cytochrome P3A4 activity
Dazao	Insomnia	A rare reaction is 'Dazao-induced angioneurotic edema'
Ephedra	As a stimulant	Currently banned in the USA and prescription only in the UK
Fuling	Insomnia, disturbed dreams	No known side-effects
Fuxiaomai	Insomnia	None unless coeliac or otherwise sensitive to gluten
Ganjiang	Insomnia	Rare – mild heartburn and GI upset

Hehuanpi	Insomnia, disturbed dreams, overarousal	Exacerbation of asthma has been reported
Hong Hwa	Insomnia	Can elevate levels of liver enzymes and white blood cells
Lingzhi	Insomnia	Minor – most commonly dry throat, nosebleeds. Can lower both blood pressure and blood sugar level. Liver damage (rare)
Longyanrou	Restless sleep, minor insomnia	Unclear
Sang Piao Xiao	Night-time enuresis	Unclear
Shouwuteng	Insomnia	None reported
Wuweizi	Insomnia, disturbed dreams, overarousal, night-time enuresis	Abdominal upset, decreased appetite and skin rash
Zhusha (cinnabar)	Night terrors	As for methyl mercury, but substantially less toxic

Appendix 5
ASSESSMENT TOOLS FOR SLEEP PROBLEMS

There are a lot of different of measures of sleep in children and adolescents. One recent review discusses 21 separate measures used in assessment (Lewandowski, Toliver-Sokol and Palermo 2011). Differences between these measures are partly because of what they are used for – some assess sleep hygiene, some sleep pattern; some are age specific while others look at specific issues like daytime sleepiness.

This table covers some of the main sleep measures and their uses. All are referred to in the text, and the key references are given to allow comparison with normative and clinical data.

Measure	Key paper/s	Uses
Sleep Diary	A variety of forms are available, one is provided below; others can be downloaded from the websites recommended at the top of page 270	Baseline in all types of sleep problem to track changes
Brief Infant Sleep Questionnaire (BISQ)	Sadeh 2004	This scale correlates well with both actigraphy and sleep diary measures
Children's Sleep Hygiene Scale (CSHS)	Harsh, Easley and LeBourgeois 2002	This is a parent-report assessment of sleep hygiene in 2–8-year-olds
Adolescent Sleep Hygiene Scale (ASHS)	LeBourgeois *et al.* 2004, 2005	An assessment of sleep hygiene in 12–17-year-olds
Adolescent Sleep-Wake Scale (AS–WS)	LeBourgeois *et al.* 2005	This assesses getting to sleep, staying asleep and sleep quality in 12–18-year-olds

Child's Sleep Habits Questionnaire (CSHQ)	Goodlin-Jones *et al.* 2008; Owens, Spirito and McGuinn 2000; Owens *et al.* 2000	A screening assessment for 4–10-year-old sleep problems, covering eight key areas: bedtime resistance sleep onset delay sleep duration sleep anxiety night-wakings parasomnias sleep-disordered breathing daytime sleepiness
Pediatric Daytime Sleepiness Scale (PDSS)	Drake *et al.* 2003	A self-report scale for 11–15-year-olds to assess EDS
Pediatric Sleep Questionnaire (PSQ)	Chervin *et al.* 2000	A parent questionnaire for 2–18-year-olds. It assesses sleep-related behaviour disorders, snoring, sleepiness and daytime behavioural issues
Epworth Sleepiness Scale (ESS)	Johns 1991	This widely used scale assesses EDS. It has adult normative data but can also help in adolescent screening
Pittsburgh Sleep Quality Index (PSQI)	Buysse *et al.* 1989; Carpenter and Andrykowski 1998	This is also an adult scale. It assesses the quality of sleep. It has comparison data on good sleepers, sleep-disordered patients and depressed patients
Children's ChronoType Questionnaire (CCTQ)	Werner *et al.* 2009	A parent report measure for use with 4–11-year-olds. It discriminates three chronotypes, and provides data that correlate with group differences on actigraphy
Flinders Fatigue Scale (FFS)	Gradisar *et al.* 2007; Hudson *et al.* 2009	This was originally an adult measure. It has more recently been used as a measure of recent fatigue in an anxious 7–12-year-old population
BEARS screening instrument	Owens and Dalzell 2005	This is a simple five-item screening tool to identify sleep problems in 2–12-year-olds
Behavioral Evaluation of Disorders of Sleep Scale (BEDSS)	Schreck 1997/1998; Schreck, Mulick and Rojahn 2003	A systematic assessment of common sleep problems – this has comparative data from 307 families of 5–12-year-olds
Bedtime Routines Questionnaire	Henderson and Jordan 2010	A sleep hygiene questionnaire for parents of 2–8-year-olds

Sleep diaries can be downloaded from various websites. Sleepforkids, which is part of the US National Sleep Foundation, has a good diary for children, at: www.sleepforkids.org/pdf/SleepDiary.pdf

A simple adult diary is produced by the Loughborough Sleep Research Centre, and can be downloaded from: www.nhs.uk/Livewell/insomnia/Documents/sleepdiary.pdf

Sleep diary

Name _____

Person recording information _____

Date _____

Age _____

Medication _____

Time	Location	Behaviour	Setting events

- *Time:* Time sleep began and time/s awakened

- *Location:* Where the person slept

- *Behaviour:* Any significant behaviours (e.g. snoring, speech, crying out, sweating)

- *Setting events:* Any relevant events (e.g. background noise, awoken by..., room unusually hot/cold)

Example sleep diary

Name: Philip Potts
Person recording information: Mrs Potts (mother)
Date: 25 November 2013
Age: 4 years 7 months
Medication: Not on any medications

Day 1

Time	Location	Behaviour	Setting events
19.15	Living room	Changed into his night-nappy and bedclothes NO ISSUES	Prompted by Mum
19.30	Bathroom	Went to the toilet and washed his face and hands, had teeth brushed DID EVERYTHING AS ASKED	Mum present, regulated water temperature, reminded him about using soap for washing
19.45	Bedroom	Settled in bed, had short story read to him, drowsy by time Mum was leaving room NO DISTRESS	Mum present until he seemed settled
21.00	Bedroom	Checked on – sleeping soundly	Nothing to note
22.30	Bedroom	Checked on – sleeping soundly	Nothing to note
23.15	Bedroom	Sitting up in bed, seems awake and very upset, not responding to cuddles or when asked what's wrong. Seems to settle and go back to sleep after about 25 minutes. Clean and dry DISTRESSED	Nothing to note. Mum stayed until he had settled
03.20	Bedroom	Pattern similar to 23.15 DISTRESSED Night-nappy saturated and needing to be changed. Settled back to sleep once changed, by 03.44	Nothing to note. Mum stayed until he had settled
07.10	Bedroom	Woke as normal, good mood, playing in bed with toys	Nothing to note

Sources for the assessment tools outlined in the table

Brief Infant Sleep Questionnaire (BISQ)
Downloadable from: www.sleep.tau.ac.il/BISQ%20-%20Pediatrics%202004.pdf

Child Sleep Hygiene Scale (CSHS)
This is a 25-item scale, with each item scored on a six-point scale from 'Never' to 'Always'. It was developed by the Sleep Research Laboratory of the University of Southern Mississippi as a parent-report measure for sleep hygiene in 2–8 year-olds. In the original paper, which presented data on 246 US children, the mean score on the scale in children without sleep issues was 57.2 (maximum possible score = 150).

Refer to the original paper for further details; the scale is reproduced below:

		1	2	3	4	5	6
1	Naps within 4 hours of bedtime						
2	Caffeine within 4 hours of bedtime						
3	Does things that are relaxing before bedtime						
4	Drinks a lot of liquids before bedtime						
5	Plays rough before bedtime						
6	Does things that are alerting before bedtime						
7	Goes to bed about the same time every day						
8	Complains of being hungry at bedtime						
9	Does things in bed that keep him/her awake						
10	Goes to bed in the same place						
11	Goes to bed feeling upset						
12	Goes to bed with worries						
13	Sleeps in a darkened room						
14	Sleeps in a room that is too hot or too cold						
15	Sleeps in a room where there are loud noises						
16	Sleeps alone (in his/her own bed)						
17	Sleeps in a room that is stuffy						
18	Sleeps all or part of the night with someone else						
19	Sleeps in a bed that is comfortable						
20	Sleeps in a home where someone smokes						
21	Has a calming bedtime routine						
22	Uses bed for things other than sleep						
23	Put to bed after falling asleep						
24	Stays up past usual bedtime						
25	Gets out of bed about same time in morning						

1: Never; 2: Occasional; 3: Sometimes; 4: Typical; 5: Frequent; 6: Always

Adolescent Sleep Hygiene Scale (ASHS)

This is a 28-item scale, with each item scored on a 6-point scale from 'never' to 'always'. Questions are clustered to cover nine specific topics: physiological, cognitive, emotional, sleep environment, daytime sleep, substance use, bedtime routine, sleep stability and bed/bedroom sharing. It has been standardised on samples of 12–17-year-old adolescents from the USA (N=552) and Italy (N=776).

The ASHS appears as an appendix to the LeBourgeois *et al.* (2005) article, and is downloadable from: http://pediatrics.aappublications.org/content/115/Supplement_1/257.full

Adolescent Sleep–Wake Scale (AS–WS)

This is a 28-item scale, with each item scored on a six-point scale from 'Never' to 'Always'. Separate groups of items deal with going to bed, falling asleep, maintaining sleep, reinitiating sleep and returning to wakefulness.

The AS–WS also appears as an appendix to the LeBourgeois *et al.* (2005) article, and is also downloadable from: http://pediatrics.aappublications.org/content/115/Supplement_1/257.full

Child's Sleep Habits Questionnaire (CSHQ) (preschool and school-age)

This is a 51-item scale. All items are scored as 'usually', sometimes' or 'rarely' and for whether or not the item is seen as a problem. Items are clustered as 'night-time', 'sleep behaviour', 'waking during the night' and 'morning waking'. It was originally standardised on 469 normal 4–10-year-old children and a sample of 154 children attending a paediatric sleep disorder clinic.

The abbreviated 22-item version of the CSHQ and a scoring document can be downloaded from: www.gse.uci.edu/childcare/pdf/questionnaire_interview/Childrens%20Sleep%20Habits%20Questionnaire.pdf

Pediatric Daytime Sleepiness Scale (PDSS)

The PDSS can be downloaded from the Iowa Sleep Disorders Center website at: www.iowasleep.com/pdfs/Pediatric%20Daytime%20Sleep iness%20Scale.pdf

The Pediatric Sleep Questionnaire (PSQ)

This 22-item scale was standardised on a sample of 54 children (age range 2–18) with polysomnographically confirmed sleep-disordered breathing, and 108 children who were attending general paediatric clinics.

This scale would need to be obtained from the source paper or by contacting the lead author, Dr Chervin. At the time of writing Dr Chervin is based at the Mayo School of Graduate Medical Education in Rochester, Maryland, USA.

Epworth Sleepiness Scale (ESS)

The original version of the ESS is available for personal use from the author's website (http://epworthsleepinessscale.com) or from the charity Narcolepsy UK at: www.narcolepsy.org.uk/about-narcolepsy/ epworth-sleepiness-scale. To enquire about licensing for clinical or commercial use contact Dr Murray Johns at:

Optalert Ltd
Level 3
Building 5
658 Church Street
Richmond
Melbourne
Victoria, 3121
Australia
Tel: +61 3 9425 5000
Fax: +61 3 9425 5001
Email: mjohns@optalert.com

or:

MAPI Research Trust
PRO Information Support
27 Rue de la villette
69003 Lyon
France
Tel: +33 (0) 4 7213 6575
Fax: +33 (0) 4 7213 6682
Email: PROinformation@mapi-trust.org

Pittsburgh Sleep Quality Index (PSQI)

This scale can be accessed through the University of Pittsburgh Sleep Medicine Institute website: www.sleep.pitt.edu/content.asp?id=1484. Copyright is owned by the university and permission for use needs to be obtained from the first author.

Children's ChronoType Questionnaire (CCTQ)

This is a 27-item scale for assessment of the typical sleep pattern in a child presenting with erratic sleep. This scale has been standardised on 152 children (77 boys, 75 girls) aged 4–11 years (mean 6.7y+1.5y).

This scale is an appendix to the source paper. This is an NIH public access manuscript and can be downloaded from: www.ncbi.nlm.nih.gov/pmc/articles/PMC2988284

Flinders Fatigue Scale (FFS)

This is a simple seven-item scale for rating daytime fatigue associated with insomnia. It is uses a five-point rating on six of the items and a seven-period rating for times of peak tiredness. Clinical use of the scale is based on an initial online validation study; a study of sensitivity to change in a five-week CBT programme for insomnia; and a study that used the scale in assessment of sleep patterns in 7–12-year-old children with clinical anxiety.

This scale is an appendix to the first source paper. The paper is a PubMed Central open access document and can be downloaded from: www.ncbi.nlm.nih.gov/pmc/articles/PMC2556916

BEARS screening instrument (adolescent questions)

This is a brief screening scale consisting of five core questions and four supplementary ones. It is not a standardised scale and is recommended for use by clinicians familiar both with the symptoms and risk factors for adolescent sleep problems.

Refer to the source paper for further information. The acronym BEARS stands for key questions about:

- Bedtime problems

- Excessive daytime sleepiness

- Awakenings during the night

- Regularity and duration of sleep

- Sleep-disordered breathing.

The supplementary questions are about daytime napping, exercise, stimulants (caffeine, tea and cola) and alcohol intake.

Behavioral Evaluation of Disorders of Sleep Scale (BEDSS)

Data using this scale has been published on 1361 5–12-year-old children. Factor analysis identified five different types of sleep issues:

- expressive sleep disturbances

- sensitivity to the environment

- disoriented awakening

- requiring sleep facilitators (medication/pacifier)

- apnoea/bruxism.

This scale was developed by Dr Kimberly Schreck, who is at the time of writing Associate Professor of Psychology at Penn State University in Harrisburg. Further information, including a list of publications, can be found at: http://harrisburg.psu.edu/faculty-and-staff/kimberly-schreck-phd

Bedtime Routines Questionnaire

This is a recent scale developed by Jill Henderson and Sara Jordan at the University of Mississippi in Harrisburg. It is a 31-item questionnaire with five-point rating on each item. The scale has four subscales, and covers weekday and weekend bedtime routines, reactivity to changes in routine, and activities before bedtime. The scale is reproduced in their paper.

Appendix 6
PREPARING FOR MEDICAL PROCEDURES

As you will have seen while going through this book, specific tests can help in clarifying the nature of the sleep problem and in working out the best way to help.

Much of what is covered in this appendix concerns assessments that are likely to be carried out in a hospital department. If you are aware that these procedures are likely to cause difficulty, help can often be obtained from the nursing or clinical psychology service in preparation for the tests themselves.

This may seem like an additional effort, but if good results can be obtained first time round, this sort of preparation may be by far the best strategy. Such help may not be routinely provided, however, and material is detailed here to enable appropriate support to be sought where needed.

A useful overview with much practical advice on helping children cope with a variety of conditions and medical procedures can be found in James Varni's old but excellent little book *Clinical Behavioural Pediatrics* (1992). This has been a ready reference and starting point for me in supporting families with many conditions over the years.

A range of methods can be used to prepare people for medical procedures. The most common is a graded approach called 'systematic desensitisation'. This involves gradually getting them used to situations that are more and more similar to the procedure, presented in increasing order of difficulty and usually paired with some form of relaxation.

Anaesthesia
What is it?
Anaesthesia is the process of administering either a local anaesthetic to make part of the body insensitive to pain during a procedure (such

as getting an injection that numbs the nerves in a tooth before having dental work carried out), or a general anaesthetic, usually given by injection or inhalation to make the person unconscious, insensitive to pain and unaware of procedures that would be difficult to carry out when they were awake.

Why might it be important?

For a number of different types of investigation, it may prove easiest for everyone if they are carried out under a general anaesthetic. This may be the best way to progress things provided that it is felt to be safe and the best way of ensuring that useful results can be obtained. Anaesthesia comes with its own issues and giving anaesthetic more frequently than needed is a risk in its own right. The anaesthetist is the appropriate professional to decide on this, weighing up factors such as likely benefits, any associated heart issues, the risk of seizures, practical issues in administering anaesthesia, the cooperation of the person being sedated, informed consent and tolerance to medications.

Sometimes when someone is put under with a general anaesthetic, this presents a good opportunity for several types of work to be carried out at the same time. Many children with ASD require a general anaesthetic to have dental work carried out, and this may provide an opportunity to do other things like taking blood samples, and possibly EEG or MRI if the procedure is carried out in a hospital setting. It can be useful to try to ensure that such studies are coordinated to carry out as much work as possible under a single procedure.

Is it simple?

This type of procedure would only be carried out in a clinic/hospital setting. The anaesthetic procedure would vary depending on the reason for doing it and any potential medical complications (such as asthma, cardiac or seizure issues). Any anaesthetic procedure would be overseen by a clinical anaesthetist and any question of possible risks would be clarified by them when obtaining informed consent.

Is it sore?

This will depend on the type of procedure and the length of time it takes to carry out.

How to prepare

Being anaesthetised can be a difficult procedure to undergo in itself. There is some evidence that simple distractions like hand-held video games used in the period before anaesthesia can reduce the build-up of anxiety beforehand and reduce anxiety after (Patel *et al.* 2006).

Where an in-dwelling butterfly line (a needle, with plastic 'wings' that can be taped to the skin to prevent it coming away and make it look a little like a butterfly, which is used to maintain medication levels during the anaesthesia) will be used to maintain anaesthesia, numbing of the skin prior to inserting the needle can be helpful, using a local anaesthetic. This is usually applied as a cream 15 minutes or so in advance to allow the anaesthetic agent to be absorbed through the skin.

Salivary melatonin testing

What is it?

This is a simple test, from three saliva samples taken at different times of day, of the profile of circulating melatonin levels.

Why might it be important?

A number of persistent sleep difficulties in ASD are 'circadian rhythm disorders' due to abnormal melatonin metabolism (Part B). This is a simple test that indicates whether someone's circulating melatonin levels are abnormal.

Is it simple?

Provided that the child is able and prepared to spit on request.

Is it sore?

No.

How to prepare

All that is required is that the child can provide the samples, which are then sealed in small vials and sent for analysis. Probably getting them to practise beforehand is the best preparation – if the person providing the saliva has limited language, demonstrating what to do and getting them to copy may be the easiest approach.

Blood draws

Having bloods taken can be uneventful, painless and simple, but is commonly traumatic, sometimes painful, and is something that many parents worry about.

What is it?

Having a needle inserted into a vein, typically in the upper arm, and a small amount of blood drawn off into a syringe to enable this to be tested.

Why might it be important?

Blood samples can be used for many types of test including genetic testing, looking at specific metabolites and identifying possible inborn errors of metabolism, amino acid profiling and essential fatty acids. Many specific differences can be linked to sleep disorders and can help to decide the best approach to management.

Is it simple?

Taking blood is usually a simple, quick process provided that the person remains relaxed and does not struggle.

Is it sore?

The procedure can be relatively painless if carried out by an experienced clinician. Some units have people (known as phlebotomists) who do nothing other than take blood samples.

As for anaesthesia, it is possible to use an anaesthetic cream to reduce pain sensation at the site where the blood draw is to be taken. If the child is distracted when the needle is inserted this often makes the procedure completely painless.

How to prepare

A number of different things can help. Some are very simple – using some novel form of distraction can be helpful. One study with 100 3.5–13-year-olds randomised them to two groups. Half of the children were distracted by looking through a kaleidoscope as a blood sample was taken while the others had a routine blood draw with no distraction (Vessey, Carlson and McGill 1994). The kaleidoscope significantly reduced the children's ratings of how distressing they found the procedure.

Possible issues

Several issues can make taking blood more difficult; these are briefly mentioned below and where known should be drawn to the attention of the clinicians planning to take the sample.

NEEDLE PHOBIA

Fear of needles is not uncommon, either in children or in adults. As many fears and phobias are passed on to children through observing the fearful reactions of adults, and often through observing their parents or grandparents, it is sensible if everyone who is going to be involved in helping and who has a fear of needles is given some help to get over this at the same time as the child.

The approach that is often most effective, as for most other monosymptomatic phobias, is some form of relaxation training followed by systematic desensitisation.

BLOOD PHOBIA

Blood phobia is also a fairly common problem. It can often interfere with a child's ability to undergo procedures such as having blood samples drawn. The important thing to realise about blood phobia is that, unlike other phobias, rather than being associated with increased autonomic arousal and elevated blood pressure, the opposite pattern is seen. People who are troubled by blood phobia typically pass out as a consequence of low blood pressure and need to be encouraged to keep their blood pressure up rather than to relax.

HEIGHTENED PAIN SENSITIVITY

Sensory functions can be acute in some people with ASD, and some will have elevated pain sensitivity. In these people, having a needle inserted could cause greater pain than normal.

Having an EEG (electroencephalograph)

What is it?

A clinical EEG is a recording of changes in brain electrical activity between pairs of scalp-mounted electrodes.

Why might it be important?

An EEG can help to identify abnormal electrical activity characteristic of epileptic activity, and be used to track the different stages seen in brain activity during sleep.

Is it simple?

The recording procedure is simple and once the electrodes are in place does not cause discomfort.

Is it sore?

In some people (myself included) it can take a little time and effort to get a good signal from the electrodes but there is no pain involved. It may take a number of washes to get all of the electrode gel out of the person's hair after the procedure.

How to prepare

Two studies have shown that simple behavioural approaches, breaking the procedure down into simple steps, with differential reinforcement (rewards for complying and cooperating with each step of the procedure) and escape avoidance can be helpful in preparing children with ASD or with other developmental issues for undergoing an EEG (see: DeMore *et al.* 2009; Slifer, Avis and Frutchey 2008).

These papers are downloadable from: www.ncbi.nlm.nih.gov/ pmc/articles/PMC2897721/pdf/nihms210820.pdf and www.ncbi. nlm.nih.gov/pmc/articles/PMC2898154/pdf/nihms210857.pdf

Having an MRI scan

What is it?

This is a common type of brain scanning procedure now available in many paediatric hospitals. Because it requires the subject to remain still for up to an hour in a confined, noisy space and sometimes requires injection of a contrast agent, it is difficult for many children to undergo without general anaesthetic.

Why might it be important?

Where there is the possibility of a structural abnormality that could be related to the presentation.

Is it simple?

The assessment itself is simple, but it is often lengthy, noisy and is difficult for children who do not tolerate confined spaces.

Is it sore?

The MRI itself is not, but the use of contrast medium requires insertion of a cannula into a vein for injection during the scan, and this can be uncomfortable.

How to prepare

One study from an Australian group has shown good results from helping the child to prepare for the scan by practising the procedure in a full-size mock-up scanner with the help of an educational play therapist (Hallowell *et al.* 2008). The preparation resulted in successful scans being obtained in the vast majority without anaesthesia. Successful scans were obtained across all ages, including in 95% of the children aged below 6. In many places younger children are routinely scanned under general anaesthetic due to the high level of difficulty in getting them to comply with the procedure.

Having an upper endoscopy

What is it?

This is a technique for examining the lining of the throat. A fibre-optic tube (called an endoscope) is used. The tube needs to be fed down into the throat through the mouth. This is an uncomfortable procedure that can induce retching and it often needs to be carried out under general anaesthetic.

Why might it be important?

Gastroesophageal reflux, where the person regurgitates stomach contents up into the throat, is a problem not uncommonly associated with sleep problems in ASD. It is caused when the flap at the top of the stomach fails to work properly. This can usually be repaired by a minor surgical procedure.

Is it simple?

The endoscopy procedure itself is simple, but it is uncomfortable, invasive, and typically needs to be carried out under a general anaesthetic.

Is it sore?

The procedure can result in bruising to the lining of the throat and make swallowing uncomfortable for a period afterwards.

How to prepare

As the process is likely to have to be carried out under anaesthetic, see the earlier section on preparing for anaesthesia.

Having an MCU (micturating cystourethrogram)

What is it?

In a MCU the bladder is filled with sterile water through a catheter and a recording is made as the bladder empties. This is used to look for any abnormality in the working of the muscles at the bladder neck that control urine retention.

Why might it be important?

This procedure might be part of the investigation for persistent night-time enuresis to exclude any constitutional basis to the problem.

Is it simple?

The assessment involves a team as it requires insertion of a catheter and visualisation of bladder emptying, usually with a real-time X-ray system.

Is it sore?

The procedure should be relatively painless and can be carried out without sedation in a cooperative person.

How to prepare

To most children an MCU will appear a bizarre and inappropriate procedure. It involves adults doing unusual things to them. The combination of providing information on the procedure (including, where appropriate, demonstration of what is involved using an anatomically correct gender-appropriate doll), coping skills training (breathing exercises and positive self-statements) and advice to parents on how to help their child can significantly reduce distress, and improve coping and cooperation (see: Phillips, Watson and MacKinlay 1998; Zelikovsky *et al.* 2000).

Appendix 7
TROUBLESHOOTING

Things don't always work out as we had hoped and with the best of intentions you might find that things have not worked as well as you had hoped. This appendix covers some of the issues that might help to pinpoint and sort out things that have prevented your approach from working according to plan.

'We already tried that – it was a complete waste of time'

You might go through the problem-solving approach covered in the book and decide that you are pretty sure what the problem is. You may think you have already tried the recommended approach to tackling it and know that nothing has improved. This is quite common by the time people seek 'professional' help. Often the more obvious solutions will already have been tried.

If all approaches were just common sense, there would be no need for a book like this, or for professionals who specialise in treating sleep problems. (For a general account of why common sense doesn't always make sense, see: Watts 2011.)

Often I see families who can run through a long list of all of the more 'common sense' approaches that they have tried but without much success.

There can be various reasons for this. Sometimes approaches that would have worked have not been stuck with for long enough to see any benefit. Sometimes approaches have been tried that work for some sorts of problem but that don't help for this particular problem. Sometimes the obvious common sense approach is just wrong and the best solution is different to what you might expect.

Why things can get worse before they get better

People are often confused when using an approach that is likely to help, but can sometimes make things even worse before they improve (this is often called an 'extinction burst'). If you have already tried a solution that seemed the right thing to do but the problem got worse, at least you know that the solution you tried had an effect on sleep. If you are convinced that you need to try this approach again, it can also help to know in advance that you may have to go through another period of poorer sleep before you start to make progress. If you gave up and the problem had deteriorated, the problem might be more treatment-resistant because of the earlier experience.

That a successful approach to sorting the problem can make things worse at first seems odd. A more obvious example might help:

▬ Imagine you have a small child, let's call him Barry. Barry tantrums when he wants ice cream. The tantrums happen when he is reminded about it, usually by the sound of an ice cream van, when going round the supermarket with his mum, or when walking past a café. The strategy sometimes works for him, particularly when his grandparents are around.

You have decided it makes sense to ignore Barry's tantrums and give him ice cream only when he is quiet and well behaved. To start with, Barry has no idea that the tantrums that often get him an ice cream no longer work, and in recent months this is the pattern that has always led up to him being bought one. For Barry, being quiet and obedient doesn't seem an obvious strategy to try when what works well is bawling his head off. Being quiet has never been rewarded with ice cream before and he doesn't expect it to happen now.

The next few times you refuse to give in to him when he hears the van approaching: You are out shopping and pass the ice cream counter in a café, or the freezer section in the supermarket, what do you think Barry will do?

It shouldn't come as too much of a surprise if Barry's tantrums seem longer and noisier than ever. *You* know your new rules but *he* doesn't; he just assumes that his 'tried and tested tantrum method' will still work – he has trained you to respond to it, and it seems to have worked pretty well up to now.

Why the books and papers aren't always right

Clinicians, researchers and their employers not surprisingly prefer to write about their successes than their failures. Somehow books and papers on things like *My greatest clinical failures* and *Experiments that didn't work out as I expected* don't get written nearly as often as *The...*

Method or *How to stop doing... the... Way*. Unless of course you believe there is a good reason why you got different results, and that that makes your view somehow better or more accurate. Even then many are reluctant to question well-accepted ideas – look what happened to Galileo. People are less prone to write up and publish 'poorer' outcomes.

If a report of a new treatment appears in the press, it has to be 'newsworthy' so will tend to be portrayed as a 'major advance' or a study that 'proves' that the approach works. There is seldom any reference to exceptions, side-effects or difficulties.

We all tend to focus on our achievements and conveniently ignore our failures – we look for the silver lining and tend to ignore the cloud. Except, that is, when we are stressed, depressed or not sleeping well, and at these times we ignore the silver lining and only see the clouds.

Academic journals can also be very picky about what they will agree to publish, wanting to focus on positive results not failures to replicate – these will also highlight the publications they appear in and strengthen their profile. This is part of the problem known as publication bias. 'Failed' studies are less likely to get published (i.e. good studies that show something has not worked) as compared to successful ones (i.e. where the treatment outcome was positive). This has recently been illustrated in research highlighting publication bias in studies on the use of medications to treat repetitive behaviour in ASD (Carrasco, Volkmar and Bloch 2012).

As publication bias favours 'successes' it weakens the chances that published papers will reflect the real chance that an approach will be of benefit – the stronger the 'cherry picking' the less representative the literature becomes. Negative studies may have been completed but be unpublished and gathering dust. They are less likely to be submitted and are more likely to be rejected when they are. In the USA and the UK funded research studies that have passed ethical review now have to be registered once they are begun, and before any results are collected. This makes it easier to track down unpublished poor results as well as locating the published results (which will usually be positive). The early fruits of this process are leading to increasing concern that publication bias has been a significant problem in the past, generating a misleadingly optimistic picture of clinical benefit (see: Denne 2012).

Many sleep problems will get better without treatment. If a problem is fairly common and is likely to improve whatever you do, a proportion of people who try a successful approach and whose sleep problems improve would have done so anyway. (Some of those on an active treatment will improve for the same reasons as a similar proportion of controls and be unrelated to any specific treatment.) They would have improved anyway.

Obviously you can never be sure if someone who has improved falls into this category (in trials they are called 'false positives') but studies can give you get an idea of the likely proportions. You need a clear understanding of how treatments are assessed to decide what works and what doesn't.

Before embarking on any approach, it is important to be as sure as you can that:

- the problem is unlikely to spontaneously and quickly get better – that you need to do something or it is likely to persist

- your chosen approach has no known significant risks – that anything you decide to do will do more good than harm

- it is likely to help – there is evidence of benefit, or that the approach at the least is plausible.

Why you can't just trust therapists because they believe in what they are doing

Most therapists carry out treatments that they believe in. Where the approach they offer is not a standard approach they are also likely to attract clients who are are more likely to believe that their less usual approach could help.

In healthcare systems run by private insurance, other factors can also come into play. Different recommendations can be made depending on how the system operates (see: Rodwin 2011). This results in marked differences between parts of the USA and between the US system and others such as those in France, Japan and the UK.

Therapists looking to attract more business may point to cases they have treated who have improved. People who have attended them are also likely to believe that any improvement has resulted from their approach. If you have sought out an expensive therapist who you believe will be able to help you, there is a strong and entirely rational incentive to believe that any improvements you see after beginning treatment are a result of the intervention you are paying for. No one would be likely to pay for a treatment they were dismissive or distrustful of, or to do something they did not believe in. Unfortunately, although believing in an effective approach is no bad thing, it is easy to believe in something that does not work.

Commercial websites may offer support to families, full of glowing comments from satisfied customers. Remember that the unsolicited comments are unlikely to be picked at random from an in-box full of such material but are more likely to be from people who are supportive of their approach. They could be from people who had been offered free treatment or other incentives. If 19 out of 20 comments are positive, unsolicited and randomly selected, this could be an excellent recommendation. It could as easily be 1 in 100 that are positive, and there is no easy way of checking.

Making sure that you are up-to-date with the evidence

When doing your background research, it is important to try to keep up-to-date. New studies and reviews of best practice appear all the time and best advice on what should be done with a given problem is bound to change. You may say 'Why should I have to do that? That's the therapist's job, I'm the parent/carer...' A good reason is that most clinicians are generalists, working daily with a wide range of referred problems in many different sorts of people. The literature is enormous and constantly growing, and few clinicians will have the time to keep fully up to date. In contrast, you are focused on one person with a specific problem. Once you know what the problem is, and you have learned how, you can probably keep up with new research and new ideas on the specific issues.

Many people, especially families of those with ASDs, prefer where possible to use complementary and alternative treatments (CAMs). Several reviews of CAMs and alternative medicine have concluded that some approaches may be of benefit (see: Aitken 2008). It is also important to know that some CAMs can have significant risks when compared to conventional alternatives (see: Kruskal 2009; Lim, Cranswick and South 2010). Because something is natural does not necessarily mean that it is always safe or safer; equally, it may be effective but have a weaker evidence base.

The difficulty in teasing out what works is the reason for the heavy reliance now being placed on 'evidence-based' practice. This emphasises where possible using treatments with good research evidence of benefit in randomised controlled trials (RCTs). This would be the ideal, but if you wait for a research group to do an adequate RCT to show whether a treatment might work you are likely to be waiting for a long time. One reason for this is the expense of conducting such research; another is that some problems and approaches are just not so easy to assess in this way.

An extreme example that illustrates why some situations don't lend themselves to this type of evidence-based approach can be found in an amusing little article reviewing the evidence that parachutes may be useful in preventing death or injury from 'gravitational challenge'. Having failed to find any RCTs on this important issue, the authors concluded:

> As with many interventions intended to prevent ill health, the effectiveness of parachutes has not been subjected to rigorous evaluation by using randomised controlled trials. Advocates of evidence-based medicine have criticised the adoption of interventions evaluated by using only observational data. We think that everyone might benefit if the most radical protagonists of evidence based medicine organised and participated in a double blind, randomised, placebo controlled, crossover trial of the parachute. (Smith and Pell 2003)

This is an extreme and tongue-in-cheek example but it illustrates the point that not every type of intervention can measure up to these criteria. The same is true of any approach that is difficult to administer without the person being treated being able to tell what is being done – speech therapy, dietary intervention – and most behavioural approaches fall into this group.

Just because there are no randomised trials does not mean that something is not true or that an approach will not work (for discussion, see: Schreck 2001).

I am fairly sure that breathing is important to maintaining human life. I don't feel it is important to carry out a randomised controlled trial to prove it and would not be prepared to take part in one. The old adage that 'absence of evidence is not evidence of absence' often holds true – there may be reasons other than lack of benefit that account for why an effective treatment has a weak evidence base.

A patentable and plausible drug therapy usually has strong financial backing because there is the anticipation of lucrative rewards for those investing in it. Research on those same effective treatments is much harder to find once a medication is off-patent and its profit margin nosedives as it has to compete against cheap generic equivalents. This can lead to the paradoxical situation where patentable treatments that are less effective can end up with stronger evidence bases than their off-patent competitors.

Those wanting to research complementary or alternative therapies usually have limited access to funding, and have a smaller pool of patients from whom to generate subjects. Even with good, positive results, there would be limited prospects of recouping the costs of any research, even if the approach were shown to be highly effective.

To keep up to date on new developments, periodically check online resources like BMJ Clinical Evidence, and the Cochrane Collaboration for the appearance of update reviews on evidence-based best practice. Various bodies like NICE (the National Institute for Clinical and Research Excellence) and SIGN (Scottish Intercollegiate Guidelines Network) periodically publish guidance on best practice – their update cycles are less frequent so may be somewhat behind those of Cochrane or BMJ Clinical Evidence reviews.

- BMJ Clinical Evidence: http://clinicalevidence.bmj.com/ceweb/index.jsp

- Cochrane Collaboration: www.thecochranelibrary.com/view/0/index.html

- National Institute for Clinical Excellence (NICE): www.nice.org.uk

- Scottish Intercollegiate Guidelines Network (SIGN): www.sign.ac.uk

A large number of papers review treatments for sleep problems. Most reviews emphasise the role of a particular type of approach, psychological or pharmaceutical interventions in the main. Here I have tried to include a range of approaches that people seem to access, rather than confining coverage only to those that may be offered through more standard health routes.

'It ain't what you do it's the way that you do it'

Sometimes there can be a 'therapist-specific effect' – a particular person seems to get good results with an approach, but the approach doesn't seem to work as well for others. This problem was discussed as early as the 1930s:

> In the hands of a limited number of individuals, virtually every method that was proposed seemed to produce cures; but the inability of other persons to obtain equally good results by what appeared to be precisely the same objective procedures eventually made it clear that the effectiveness of these methods was more a function of subtle psychological influences than of the particular physical praxis involved. (Mowrer and Mowrer 1938)

Unless they are still in practice, affordable, available and happen to live locally, you may be impressed, but you don't want to know that their therapy had a good result in one clinic or case that has been highly publicised (but happens to be, say, in Tucson, Arizona) or that their approach apparently gets good results but only when carried out by them. What you want to know is whether it has been effective when compared against others who had the same problem but didn't get the same treatment, and ideally that this effect has been repeated by different therapists in different places. The evidence seldom turns out to be as strong as this. In this book, I have tried to provide a review of what has been done and/or key sources that can be used to follow up any more recent evidence.

INDEX

metabolic syndrome 144, 197, 198, 204, *226, 227, 235, 238*
metabolism and visual impairments 191–192
methylphenidate 132, 133, 139, 149, *221, 223, 239*
mianserin 260
midazolam 109, *237*
modafinil 129, 130, 132, 133, 134, 149, 150, 154, 155, *228, 240*, 260
MSLT (Multiple Sleep Latency Test) 147, *220*
mu rhythm 192, *233, 237*
myotonic dystrophy 127, *233*

N-acetylserotonin 191, 195, 196
narcolepsy 9, 36, 97, 127, 129, 135, 147–150, 155, 170, 179, 202, *217, 218, 221, 222, 223, 224, 230, 231, 232, 233, 234, 235, 237, 241, 243, 244*, 248, 249, 260, 274
  approaches 149
  definition 147–148
  frequency 148
  in a nutshell 150
  outcomes 149–150
Narcolepsy Association UK (UKAN) 248
Narcolepsy Network 248
National Center on Sleep Disorders Research 249
National Foundation for Sleep and Related Disorders in Children (NFSRDC) 249
National Sleep Foundation 249
neurobiology of sleep
  normal patterns of sleep 184–188
  normal range of sleep 184–188
  sleep stages 167–173
neuropeptide Y 192, 211
nightmares 9, 36, 42, 46, 60, 61, 62, 67, 69, 103–108, 109, 135, 154, 168, 171, 211, *219, 224, 227, 229, 230, 233, 236, 246*, 260
  approaches 105–107
  definition 104
  frequency 104–105
  in a nutshell 108
  outcomes 107–108
night sweats 262, 266

night terrors (a.k.a. sleep terrors; pavor nocturnus) 9, 46, 67, 104, 108–110, 123, 154, 168, 200, 212, *224, 229, 231, 234, 235, 237, 241, 246*, 262, 267
  approaches 109–110
  definition 108
  frequency 109
  in a nutshell 110
  outcomes 110
night-time eating disorders (night eating syndrome (NES) and sleep-related eating disorder (SRED)) 9, 134–137
  approaches 136
  definition 135
  frequency 135–136
  in a nutshell 137
  outcomes 136–137
nociceptive trigeminal inhibition (NTI) 140, 212
nocturia 113
nocturnal enuresis (bedwetting) 9, 111–122
  approaches 113–120
  behavioural interventions 113–117
    dry bed training (DBT) 115–116
    enuresis alarms 116–117, *224*, 252–256
    retention control training (RCTr) 114–115
  definition 111–112
  desmopressin acetate (DDAVP) 118, 122, 155
  frequency 112
  in a nutshell 122
  outcomes 120
  tricyclics 117
nocturnal frontal lobe epilepsy (NFLE) 89, *235*
nocturnal seizures 9, 82, 87–90, 104, 155, *218, 220, 235*, 256, 261
  approaches 89
  definition 87–88
  frequency 88
  in a nutshell 90
  outcomes 89–90
non-compliance 22

CPI Antony Rowe
Eastbourne, UK
December 02, 2022